DERAILED

Living with Fibrosing Mediastinitis

T J Askren, RN, BSN

The information provided in this book is designed to provide helpful information on the subjects discussed. This book is not meant to be used, nor should it be used, to diagnose or treat any medical condition. For diagnosis or treatment of any medical problem, consult your own physician. The publisher and author are not responsible for any specific health or allergy needs that may require medical supervision and are not liable for any damages or negative consequences from any treatment, action, application or preparation, to any person reading or following the information in this book. References are provided for informational purposes only and do not constitute endorsement of any websites or other sources. Readers should be aware that the websites listed in this book may change.

Red Treehouse Publishing
Red Treehouse Publishing
PO BOX 1459
Talent, OR 97540
Derailedfm.com
ISBN-13: 978-1479306374
ISBN-10: 1479306371

Acknowledgements

I'd like to thank the following people without whom I would not be writing this book:

My parents, Larry and Joanne Askren, for being by my side every moment, being my advocates, and for helping me to fight this disease.

My partner, Monica Wandro, for her love, care, and helping me to enjoy ten years of adventures.

My brother, Sean Askren, my sister, Bobi Jo Whitinger, my nieces, Brandi and Lauren Whitinger, and my nephew, Nick Askren.

My cousin, Ann Hardin, for her love and support always.

My aunt and uncle, Beverly and Gordon Butler, for visiting me in Cleveland and teaching me that living was my only option.

Michael Bain, M.D., Kim Kerr, M. D., John Liming, M.D., and Abraham Rothman, M.D. for their skills and expertise. Without them I would not be here today.

Renee, RN at Children's Heart Center in Las Vegas.

The wonderful nurses at Bethesda North Hospital in Cincinnati, UCSD in San Diego, and Sunrise Hospital in Las Vegas, for all their skill and compassion.

Sharon Banschbach, RN, for her research assistance and for encouraging me to write this book.

Lori Bonner, Mary Burrell, Bill Coffield, Sheila Durham, Tricia Edgell, Angela England, Mary Catherine Fountain, Shane Goodman, Kristina Jill Hall, Luke Hall, Brenda Humphries, Jeanieann Marie Langston-Janis, Mary Ellen Kovaleski, Richard Maples, David Martin, Melissa McMurray, Terry Palmer, Felicia Quinn, Mark Dalton Thompson, Carolyne Valaitis, and Brenda Dee Wood, for sharing their individual stories.

For Sheila and Michaela

Foreword

During the writing of this book, I was made aware of a young girl named Michaela. I didn't know Michaela personally, but found out about her through the news.

Michaela was a bright and loving young woman who played soccer and hoped to one day become a pediatrician. She lived in Minnesota and would have been a junior in high school in the fall of 2012.

Michaela's life was cut short suddenly on July 1, 2012 when she collapsed while jogging along the bike trail near her home. Believing she had been stricken with heat exhaustion, paramedics took her to the hospital where she subsequently died.

Michaela's parents were unconvinced that the heat had caused their daughter's demise and felt that there was something wrong with Michaela even before her untimely death. She had been having breathing issues for four years and, for the past three years, had been treated for asthma. In April, Michaela was diagnosed with vocal cord dysfunction, but it was unlikely that VCD caused her death.

After two long months, her parents' suspicions were confirmed. Michaela died from a cardiac arrest that was brought on by *coronary artery vasculitis*. The medical examiner discovered the real cause of Michaela's health problem: Fibrosing Mediastinitis (FM) from a histoplasmosis infection, a fungal disease that primarily attacks the lungs.

Time and time again I hear stories of people being misdiagnosed, often going through years of tests and useless treatments before they are diagnosed with fibrosing mediastinitis. Many people present with a chronic respiratory infection and are treated with antibiotics. Asthma is also a common misdiagnosis.

I have had the opportunity to meet several people with fibrosing mediastinitis. Many of them either grew up or lived in an area of the United States known to be endemic for Histoplasmosis, primarily the Ohio and Mississippi Valleys. Their ongoing respiratory infections were treated with antibiotics, in most cases, but when they failed to respond to the treatment, no further evaluation was done. It is not until they develop complications of fibrosing mediastinitis that histoplasmosis is discovered to be the cause of their earlier health problems. Most likely, most of these earlier respiratory infections were Histoplasmosis infections that could have been treated and, perhaps, prevented the development of FM.

If a patient who lives in an endemic area and exhibits symptoms of a respiratory infection that does not respond to traditional treatment, then the possibility of Histoplasmosis should be considered. In fact, over 80% of people living in endemic areas are exposed to Histoplasmosis. A prudent, aware physician will consider Histoplasmosis in patients who present with ongoing respiratory infections that do not respond to antibiotics.

I am a registered nurse. I have been working in the field of critical care and emergency/trauma medicine for 27 years. It is not within my scope of practice to diagnose disease, recommend treatment or explain potential risks and benefits of any treatments. Diagnosis and treatment of fibrosing mediastinitis and other diseases is limited to physicians. I encourage my patients to educate themselves about their diseases processes. It is imperative that we take control and responsibility of our lives and health.

Note: Any word that is in *italics* can be found in the glossary at the end of the book.

"You have Fibrosing Mediastinitis"

When I heard these words for the first time I had no idea what was being said. I had never heard of fibrosing mediastinitis. I had been in the health care field seventeen years when I was diagnosed and was completely taken aback by what the doctor told me. The physicians who were taking care of me at the time did not offer much of an explanation, nor did they offer much hope.

Let me start with the common explanation for fibrosing mediastinitis:

> *Fibrosing mediastinitis, also known as sclerosing mediastinitis or mediastinal fibrosis, is a disorder characterized by an excessive fibrotic reaction in the mediastinum. It can result in compromise of airways, great vessels, and other mediastinal structures, with morbidity directly related to the location and extent of fibrosis. Fibrosing mediastinitis is usually a sequel of histoplasmosis.*[i]

According to Dr. James Loyd, Professor of Medicine at Vanderbilt University and a respected authority on fibrosing mediastinitis, there are "at least two different syndromes of fibrosing mediastinitis (FM) that can be distinguished from other mediastinal disorders. The vast majority of FM in the United States (>90%) occurs as a late consequence of a *Histoplasma capsulatum* infection (post-histoplasmosis FM, or post-Histo FM) and is characterized by obstruction of central vessels and airways by proliferative tissue, usually containing *ectopic* calcification.

Another type, idiopathic proliferative fibrosing mediastinitis (IPFM), is a rare disorder that is characterized by extensive mediastinal proliferation *without calcification* and may affect additional extrathoracic (*outside the chest cavity)* sites concomitantly. The term "idiopathic" is medical-speak for "we don't know what the heck caused it." Many synonyms for FM have been used; including mediastinal fibrosis or sclerosing mediastinitis, but fibrosing mediastinitis is now the preferred term."[ii]

Dr. Loyd also points out that there is condition known as *mediastinal granuloma* that can be caused by Histoplasmosis, but is distinguished from FM because it is not as invasive and its outcome is more favorable.

Mediastinal granuloma is the abnormal enlargement of mediastinal lymph nodes by granulomatous inflammation, is usually asymptomatic or minimally symptomatic, and is often detected on chest radiographs taken for other reasons. The mediastinal granuloma consists of encapsulated caseous lymph nodes that are easily removed surgically.[iii]

Dr. Loyd points out that fibrosing mediastinitis is NOT just scarring in the mediastinum, but must also involve obstruction of vessels and/or airways with the absence of cancer or emboli causing the obstruction.

Ninety percent of fibrosing mediastinitis is classified as post-Histoplasmosis. Eighty percent of those have unilateral (one-sided) involvement, usually on the right side.

Ok, well, what the heck does that mean? How did I get it and what should I expect? There are a lot of words in there that I don't quite understand. What is fibrosing? What is a mediastinum? And what is Histoplasmosis?

Most people who are given this diagnosis feel as if someone snapped off the lights, leaving them floundering and bewildered. Fear and frustration are common. We fear the unknown and we are frustrated at the lack of information and medical resources. There are thousands and thousands of rare diseases. Everyone who is affected by a rare disease wants to have their condition recognized. This book focuses on one rare disease: Fibrosing Mediastinitis. It is my hope that this book can help you see some light again.

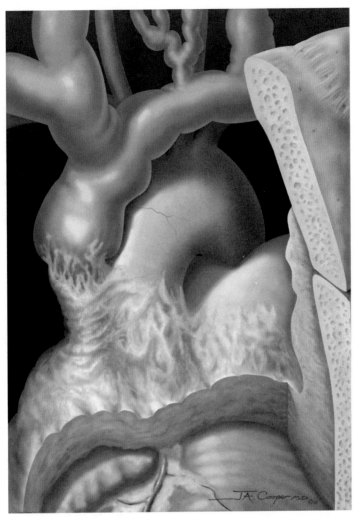

Artist's Rendition of Fibrosing Mediastinitis James A. Cooper, MD, Radiology Group, San Diego, California

What is Histoplasmosis?
Don't You Get that from Bird Poop?

Well, yes. And, no.

Histoplasmosis was first discovered in 1905 by a physician named Samuel Taylor Darling who was on a mission in Panama to curb the outbreaks of yellow fever and malaria that were wiping out the canal workers. Darling discovered strange lung granulomas in three different autopsied canal workers thought to have tuberculosis. These patients had not exhibited the typical symptoms of the other tropical diseases. Darling isolated an organism from these granulomas and, upon examining it, declared it to be a form of protozoan surrounded by a clear rim or capsule. He dubbed the organism *Histoplasmosis capsulatum* and the disease became known as Darling's Disease. Since the disease did not kill all of its hosts, it fell by the wayside, in terms of study, in the medical community. It wasn't until 1912 when a pathologist named Henrique da Rocha-Lima compared Darling's specimens to another organism that caused a disease in horses and found that *Histoplasmosis capsulatum* was actually a fungus.

H. capsulatum is found in soils throughout the world. In the United States, the fungus is endemic in the Ohio, Missouri and Mississippi Valleys. Significant populations of people with FM have had contact with these areas. The fungus, which is already in the soil, seems to thrive in soil rich in nitrogen, especially those contaminated with bird or bat droppings. The organism is not present in the bird droppings themselves. Birds do not carry or spread the disease. In contrast, bats can become infected and transmit histoplasmosis through their droppings, which is why Histoplasmosis is sometimes called splelunker's lung or cave disease.

Contaminated soil can be infected for years and outbreaks of Histoplasmosis have been associated with construction, renovation, or anything that may disturb the soil and cause the spores to become airborne.

Histoplasma capsulatum is a dimorphic fungus that remains in a vegetative form at ambient temperatures and grows as yeast at body temperature in mammals. The spores of *H. capsulatum*, that are prevalent in the soil in endemic areas, are inhaled. The spores are then ingested by the lung cells and converted into yeast. This usually occurs within 15-18 hours after exposure. The yeast cells attach to the lymph nodes. An adaptive immune response is set up within 1-2 months which shuts down further infection. This response leaves residual findings of small lung nodules and calcifications in the lung, liver and spleen. This is NOT fibrosing mediastinitis. These areas may show up incidentally on radiographs, but cause no ill effects to the person.

Histoplasmosis is the most common fungal infection in the United States. Each year, 250,000 people are found to have Histoplasmosis. In the late 1950's, after studying the organisms in patients in tuberculosis sanitariums, Dr. Michael L. Furcolow found that many of those patients actually had histoplasmosis as opposed to tuberculosis. As Medical Director of the U.S. Public Health Service field station in Kansas City, Missouri, he told the Missouri State Medical Association, in 1962, that many of the flu-like illnesses seen that summer were probably cases of histoplasmosis.

Biology of Histoplasmosis

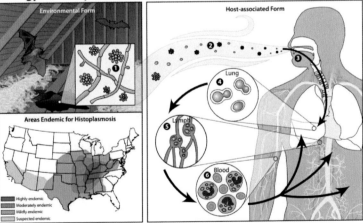

Many people who acquire Histoplasmosis never develop symptoms. Symptoms can occur anywhere from a couple of days to a few weeks and include fever, chills, dry cough, chest pain, muscle pain, headache, joint pain, and loss of appetite. Often, people mistake it for the flu. The elderly, very young or those with poor immune systems, such as people with HIV or those taking immune suppressive medications, may have more serious symptoms. The illness is not contagious.

Histoplasmosis can be diagnosed in different ways. A biopsy of affected tissue is most helpful as the spores can be readily identified. Secondly, the fungus can be cultured in 1-2 weeks. Dr. Joseph Wheat, Professor of Indiana University School of Medicine, recognized a protein of the fungus that can be detected in serum (blood) or urine. Finally, an antibody test recognizes the immune response to the fungus, but it is not specific for acute infection. [iv]

Mild cases of Histoplasmosis are not treated medically. In more severe cases, histo is treated with anti-fungal medications such as oral itraconazole or intravenous Amphotericin-B.

A critical manifestation of respiratory histoplasmosis is Acute Respiratory Distress Syndrome (ARDS), a life-threatening lung condition that prevents the exchange of oxygen in the lungs. The lungs accumulate fluid causing them to be heavy and noncompliant. It is also called stiff lung or shock lung. People with ARDS usually require *intubation* and positive end expiratory pressure (PEEP) ventilation with a breathing machine. Cases of ARDS have occurred in patients who are *immunocompromised* and in people who have been exposed to a large amount of spores. A third of ARDS patients die and survivors often have residual lung problems and/or brain injury from the effects of long-term oxygen deprivation.

Other Complications of Histoplasmosis

Fibrosing mediastinitis is the least common and most serious complication of Histoplasmosis, but it is not the only complication. Therefore, it is possible that people with post-Histo FM could have complications, not related to their FM, but to their previous Histoplasmosis infection.

Disseminated Histoplasmosis

If the histoplasmosis infection is not confined to the lungs it is referred to as *disseminated histoplasmosis*. Disseminated histoplasmosis usually only occurs in individuals who are already immunocompromised (very young, elderly, HIV+) or are exposed to a large amount of the spores. One third of cases have occurred in infants. Major risk factors include exposure to the fungus as an infant, AIDS with a low T-cell count, use of *corticosteroids*, hematologic malignancy, and solid organ transplantation. It occurs in 1 in 2000 cases of active histoplasmosis infections.

Other symptoms of disseminated histoplasmosis include gastrointestinal distress that may produce diarrhea and abdominal pain. Cardiac involvement resulting in valvular disease and cardiac insufficiency has also been reported. Histoplasmosis may produce *dyspnea*, peripheral edema, angina, and fever. Central nervous system involvement may produce headache, visual and gait disturbances, confusion, seizures, altered consciousness, and neck stiffness or pain.

Cardiac

There have been cases of histoplasmosis causing pericarditis. Pericarditis is the inflammation of the protective sac (pericardium) that surrounds the heart. This is usually due to an inflammatory response of the surrounding lymph nodes that affect the pericardium rather than from the Histoplasmosis infection itself. During two separate outbreaks of Histoplasmosis in Indiana that involved 435 cases, Dr. Wheat reported 45 cases of histo-related pericarditis.[v]

Pericarditis can cause stabbing chest pain that may worsen with deep breathing or reclining. Fever, chills, and a general ill feeling may accompany pericarditis. It is typically diagnosed using echocardiography.

Pericarditis is usually treated with non-steroidal anti-inflammatory medications, such as ibuprofen. Sometimes it is necessary to utilize short-term narcotic pain medications.

In some cases pericarditis may lead to a serious constrictive complication called *cardiac tamponade*. It is caused when the lining of the heart fills with fluid to the point that it prohibits the heart from beating effectively. The pressure must be released emergently, usually with the use of a long needle to drain the pericardial sac. In severe or recurrent cases, the pericardial sac may have to be removed surgically. This procedure is called a *pericardiectomy*.

Ocular

Presumed ocular histoplasmosis syndrome (POHS) is a distinct condition that is characterized by scarring of the vascular area of the eye between the retina and sclera (choroid) as well as the retina itself. It may also cause damage to the area of the retina known as the macula. In most cases there is no residual damage, but POHS may cause permanent visual changes or blindness. [vi]

Endocrine

The adrenal glands are two small endocrine glands situated above the kidney. Each adrenal gland has an outer cortex, which produces corticosteroids (steroid hormones), and an inner medulla, which produces norepinephrine and epinephrine (adrenaline).

Corticosteroids include hydrocortisone (cortisol), a hormone that helps the body utilize fats, proteins, and carbohydrates. They help to maintain the body's blood sugar. Corticosterone, another hormone produced by the adrenal cortex, helps suppress inflammatory reactions in the body. Aldosterone, a hormone that helps regulate blood pressure, is also produced by the adrenal cortex.

The adrenal medulla also produces hormones that help the body cope with stressful situations by increasing blood pressure and blood flow to the muscles, heart and brain.

Cases of disseminated Histoplasmosis causing adrenal masses and dysfunction (adrenal insufficiency) have been reported. Symptoms can be vague and mimic other diseases. They include progressive fatigue, muscle weakness, weight loss, and loss of appetite. Nausea, vomiting, diarrhea, dizziness, changes in blood pressure, heart rate, blood sugar problems, salt craving, and headaches are also symptoms of adrenal insufficiency. It is not to say that people having these symptoms have adrenal insufficiency, as these symptoms could be manifested by any number of disorders. The most common tool for diagnosing adrenal insufficiency is the ACTH (cosyntropin) stimulation test which is a series of blood tests to see how well the body produces cortisol.[vii]

Neurological

Meningitis is an inflammation of the membrane lining the brain and spinal cord. There have been rare cases of disseminated histoplasmosis causing meningitis. Patients exhibit symptoms of mental status changes, headaches, fever, and cranial nerve palsies, especially involving the oculomotor, abducens, and facial nerves.

Histoplasmosis meningitis is treated with the intravenous antifungal Amphotericin-B. [viii]

Skeletal

In an Indianapolis study by Dr. Jerome Rosenthal involving 381 patients during a histoplasmosis outbreak showed that just over six percent had arthritic symptoms, mostly in the knees, ankles, wrists, and small joints of the hands. A majority of these patients had mild symptoms that resolved spontaneously or with a treatment of anti-inflammatory medications. [ix]

A rare condition called mycotic arthritis, where the fungus actually settles in the joints, may become permanent if the infection is not treated with antifungal medications in its acute phase.

Studies have also shown that people with already existing rheumatoid conditions, such as rheumatoid arthritis, are at greater risk for developing infections, including histoplasmosis.

What is a Mediastinum?

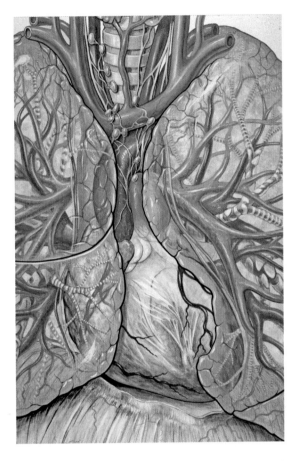

    The *mediastinum* is not a structure, but rather a space in which other structures are situated. It's a rather small space, encompassed by the lungs on each side, the sternum (breastbone) in front and the vertebral column (backbone) in the back. As you can see, it's quite crowded in the mediastinum. It may look like random mess to most people, but it's actually fairly organized. It's filled with vital structures: the heart and its many complex vessels, the trachea (windpipe) and airways to the lungs, as well as the esophagus (the gullet). The tiny bean-like structures that weave through the mediastinum, as well as the rest of the body, are called *lymph nodes*. Lymph nodes are part of the lymphatic system, a network of glands and fluid that collect and eliminate invaders, such as bacteria and fungi. The lymphatic system is essential to our immune system and our ability to fend off disease.

Most people don't know about their mediastinum. They've never even heard of a mediastinum. This is one of many reasons that people who are diagnosed with fibrosing mediastinitis are so puzzled. They are told they have a disease of something they didn't even know they had!

Symptoms of Histo-FM

Patients with Histo-FM often report symptoms for several years prior to diagnosis. Imaging reveals that the proliferative tissue usually contains heavy calcification. These symptoms are induced by the invasion of mediastinal structures and typically include, but not limited to:

- o Chest pain
- o Chest pain that worsens with breathing
- o Shortness of breath,
- o Cough
- o Coughing up blood (hemoptysis)
- o Difficult or painful swallowing
- o Dizziness
- o Syncope
- o Palpitations

There are certain criteria for a diagnosis of Histo-FM. Dr. Loyd explains the key piece to an FM diagnosis:

Heavy ectopic calcification in a proliferative mediastinal lesion causing major vascular or airway occlusion, in the absence of other conditions such as known malignancy or emboli, is sufficiently characteristic such that a biopsy is not needed for diagnosis in most cases.[x]

Diagnostic Tools

X-Rays (Radiographs)

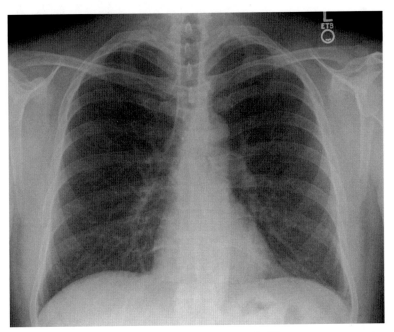

Chest x-rays are usually normal. The most common diagnostic tools for the detection of FM are the following:

Computed Tomography (CT)

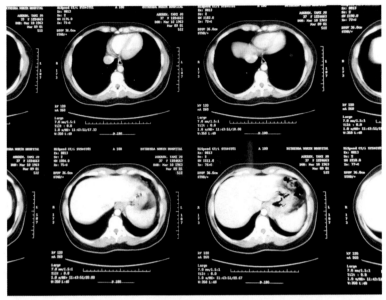

Calcifications can be seen more readily than with plain x-ray. With the use of intravenous dye, more structures and occlusions can be evaluated in cases of FM.

Also known as a CAT scan, computerized tomography is a specialized x-ray machine used to view a body part in a more detailed way. The images produced are typically cross-sectioned. That is, it gives the physician a view as if he sliced you liked deli meat and looked at each slice. This is the most common way fibrosing mediastinitis is diagnosed.

The CT is relatively painless. Sometimes a test may require an intravenous line to be placed in your arm so that the technician can inject a special dye. This is useful when the physician wants to see blood flow thorough a particular area. When this is done the procedure is called a CT Angiogram. The use of computerized tomography (CT) in the diagnosis of FM has been crucial.

Left Lung		Right Lung
59462.5	Total Counts	469100.2
11.2	Percent	88.8
6.9	1 Subregion % 4	26.1
3.4	2 Subregion % 5	56.3
0.9	3 Subregion % 6	6.3

Lung Distribution

askren
ID: 001
Acq: 12
Planar
Tc-99m
Acq Mat
Collimat
Mag: 1.0
File: R1
Image I
Acq ID:
Slice: 2
Uin: 96.
Bethesda
Cincinna

post

Left Lung		Right Lung
43867.8	Total Counts	473157.5
8.5	Percent	91.5
2.6	1 Subregion % 4	11.0
4.5	2 Subregion % 5	48.9
1.4	3 Subregion % 6	31.5

This perfusion scan shows blood filling the right lung, but very little blood filling the left lung

Nuclear Medication Scans

The most common nuclear medicine scan is the ventilation/perfusion scan (V/Q). Some people refer to it as simply a lung scan. It is helpful in evaluation of blood and air flow to the lungs. It is also helpful to determine if more than one lung is affected.

"Nuclear medicine uses very small amounts of radioactive materials (radiopharmaceuticals) to diagnose and treat disease. In imaging, the radiopharmaceuticals are detected by special types of cameras that work with computers to provide very precise pictures about the area of the body being imaged. In treatment, the radiopharmaceuticals go directly to the organ being treated. The amount of radiation in a typical nuclear imaging procedure is comparable with that received during a diagnostic x-ray, and the amount received in a typical treatment procedure is kept within safe limits."[xi]

The procedure is relatively painless, but can be uncomfortable with people with breathing problems. The patient will sit or lie down for the test. An intravenous line is placed. The test has two parts: the ventilation and the perfusion.

During the ventilation portion of the test a technician will give you a mouthpiece or a mask and ask you to breathe in a colorless odorless gas containing the radiopharmaceutical. As you breathe the gas the technician will take a series of pictures that will show the lungs' ability to take in air.

The second part of the test involves the injection of the radiopharmaceutical into an intravenous line. Again, the technician takes a series of pictures that will show the blood flow into the lungs. This test is particularly useful for those with FM because it can show where blockages occur in the major blood vessels between the heart and lungs.

Echocardiography

The very high frequency range of sound that is inaudible to the human ear is known as ultrasound. These sound waves can be used to bounce off a solid object and be translated into an image. Ultrasound has been used by the Navy to detect submarines and is also used by fishermen to find fish.

The use of ultrasound on the heart is called echocardiography (cardiac echo or simply "echo"). The test allows the physician to look at the structure of the heart, the integrity of the valves and also to evaluate for abnormal pressures in the heart chambers. He/she can also see how well the heart is pumping. If you have FM, your doctor may use this to evaluate you for *pulmonary hypertension.*

Echocardiography is painless, safe, and requires no special preparation.

Magnetic Resonance Imaging (MRI)

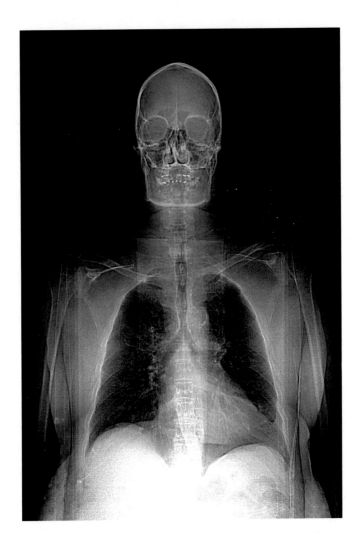

From time to time, your physician may order an MRI of your chest, but this is not standard. Most FM can be diagnosed with a CT scan.

An MRI (or magnetic resonance imaging) scan is a radiology technique that uses magnetism, radio waves, and a computer to produce images of body structures. The MRI scanner is a tube surrounded by a giant circular magnet. The patient is placed on a moveable bed that is inserted into the magnet. The magnet creates a strong magnetic field that aligns the protons of hydrogen atoms, which are then exposed to a beam of radio waves. This spins the various protons of the body producing a faint signal that is detected by the receiver portion of the MRI scanner. The receiver information is processed by a computer, and a detailed image is produced.[xii]

If you have an MRI, a technician will ask you a series of questions. Anyone having an MRI cannot have any metal in their bodies, such as aneurysm clips, prosthetics, certain types of heart valves, or shrapnel because of the strong magnet that is used.

People with claustrophobia or who have problems lying flat for long periods of time may also have difficulty with an MRI. You are placed, headfirst, into a long tube, which can be disconcerting for some people. However, the use of an "open MRI" is becoming more popular. MRI's usually take a long time to complete and can be very noisy.

Biopsy

Biopsy is a procedure, usually performed by a surgeon or radiologist, to obtain tissues and cells from a suspicious area. It often requires going into an operating room and may also require the use of general anesthesia.

General anesthesia refers to being put into a deep sleep, using medications, by a specialist called an anesthesiologist. Because this deep sleep renders you unable to move, he/she will insert a plastic breathing tube called an endotracheal tube while you are asleep to help you breathe. After surgery, the anesthesiologist will administer medications to reverse the effects of the drugs that put you to sleep. The endotracheal tube is usually removed before you completely wake up.

Biopsy is seldom useful or even safe in cases of FM. The risks of hemorrhage due to the development of collateral circulation and vascular involvement are substantial.

Angiography (Vascular Catheterization)

This may also be referred to as simply a catheterization or a cath. The use of vascular catheterization is the gold standard for evaluation of FM vascular invasion. It also affords access to the vessel for interventional mechanisms, such as *stents*, cylinder-shaped mesh medical devices that are inserted into a narrowed blood vessel to help hold the vessel open, improving blood flow.

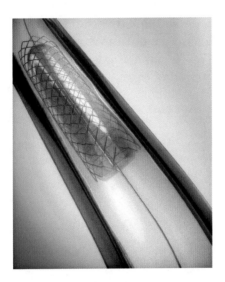

A stent inside a vessel

The procedure is done by a specialized cardiologist (heart specialist) or radiologist in a room called the cardiac catheterization lab (cardiac cath lab, or simply "cath lab"). These doctors are called interventionalists.

Depending on the procedure and the physician, the patient may be put into a light sleep or given general anesthesia. The interventionalist will make a tiny incision in the large artery in the groin (femoral artery). Some doctors prefer to use an artery in the arm. Then he/she will pass a thin wire into the artery and up through the aorta (the large "trunk" artery that passes through your body and branches off to the rest of your body) until it reaches the heart. The doctor will watch this under a special x-ray called a fluoroscope. When the catheter tip reaches the area of evaluation he/she will inject a special dye through the catheter so that the flow of blood can be seen.

If a vessel is narrow, the interventionalist will attempt to open the vessel with a balloon (angioplasty) or a stent. The stent is compressed down as it is inserted through the catheter. When the physician is satisfied with the placement, he/she opens the stent up. The catheter is withdrawn and the stent is left in the vessel.

After the procedure it is necessary for the patient to lie in bed for a minimum of six hours with his/her leg kept perfectly straight. Some people think this is the worst part of an angiogram. Because the doctor entered through an artery, the risk of bleeding is significant and it is crucial for the artery to seal itself off for a period of time.

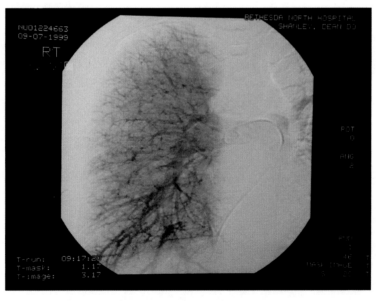

Normal right lung pulmonary angiography

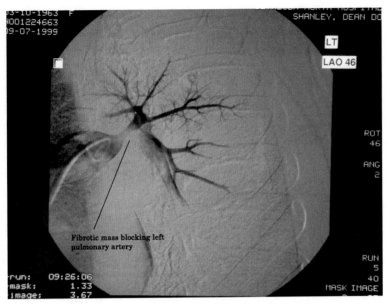

Pulmonary angiography of left lung showing dramatic stenosis and diminished blood flow to the left lung

Bronchoscopy

A bronchoscopy is a visual examination of the airways to the lungs, called the bronchi, and the smaller airways inside the lungs, called the bronchioles. You may be given sedation through an intravenous line and the doctor may use a liquid anesthetic to help numb the airways. He/she then inserts a thin flexible tube with a tiny camera on the end through your nose or mouth, down your throat and into the airways. This can cause some initial gagging and coughing. If there is a lot of bleeding in the lungs, the physician will use a larger, more rigid tube, under general anesthesia, and will pass the scope through your mouth.

During the exam the doctor can perform the following diagnostic procedures:

A Bronchoalveolar lavage. For this method, your doctor passes a small amount of saline solution (salt water) through the bronchoscope and into part of your lung. He or she then suctions the salt water back out. The fluid picks up cells and bacteria from the airway, which your doctor can study.

Transbronchial lung biopsy. For this method, your doctor inserts forceps into the bronchoscope and takes a small tissue sample from inside the lung.

Transbronchial needle aspiration. For this method, your doctor inserts a needle into the bronchoscope and removes cells from the lymph nodes in your lungs. These nodes are small, bean-shaped masses. They trap bacteria and cancer cells and help fight infections.[xiii]

Mediastinoscopy

A mediastinoscopy is a surgical procedure that requires general anesthesia whereby a thoracic surgeon or trained pulmonologist makes an incision at the top of your *sternum* and can use a tube with a camera, called a mediastinoscope, to explore the middle chest cavity. He can also perform some surgeries and take tissue samples for biopsy.

As with any surgical procedure, there are risks that your surgeon should discuss with you. They include:

- Bleeding
- Infection
- Temporary or permanent paralysis of the laryngeal nerve, which may cause hoarseness
- Pneumothorax. Collapse of the lung, causing air to become trapped in the pleural space.
- Subcutaneous emphysema (air under the skin)
- Perforation of the esophagus (hollow, muscular tube used in swallowing), trachea (windpipe), or large blood vessels of the heart is rare[xiv]

Where does the Fibrosis Come From?

Fibrosing mediastinitis is rare. Dr. L. Joseph Wheat estimates that over 500,000 people are infected with Histoplasmosis per year and over 80 percent of people living in the endemic areas have positive skin tests for Histoplasma. However, less than 1 percent of these patients with Histoplasmosis develop fibrosing mediastinitis.[xv]

Don't you wish you'd played the lottery now?

It is unclear to researchers why a small percentage of people develop FM, but the most prevalent theory is that they may have an overactive immune system.

Your immune system is responsible for identifying and fighting off foreign invaders to your body, such as bacteria, viruses, fungi, and other substances that may threaten your health. An invader may be living, such as a bacterium or a virus, or non-living, such as a chemical. An invader produces substances called *antigens*. Your body also produces its own antigens, *called human leukocyte antigens (HLAs)* which keep the body from attacking its normal cells and tissues.

Your body has several weapons in its arsenal for immunity. One is your *innate immunity* which includes skin, mucus membranes, and the ability to sneeze and cough. Your skin is the largest barrier against invaders. A cough is a reflex that the body uses to protect itself from some invaders.

We also have *acquired immunity* that we develop just by living in the world and being exposed to billions of potential invaders. Your body learns which of these invaders are harmful and which are not.

Your white blood cells (called leukocytes) are your blood's warrior cells. A type of white blood cell called a *lymphocyte* directly fights an antigen by attaching to it or by releasing a chemical to destroy it. These chemicals are known as *antibodies*.

This response in your body is called the *immune response* or inflammation. It is part of our innate immunity. When invaders cause damage to cells and tissues, the cells release chemicals to set up this response. Blood vessels leak fluid into the tissues causing swelling that help to trap the invaders and keep them from spreading to other parts of the body. Lymph nodes act as filters or traps for foreign particles and are important in the proper functioning of the immune system. They are packed tightly with the white blood cells called lymphocytes.

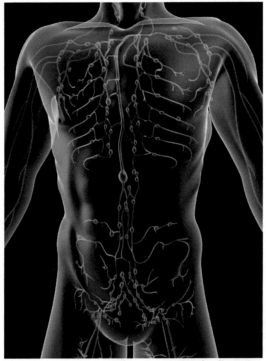

The Lymphatic System

FM is believed to be caused by an *excessive* immune response to an infection that involved the mediastinal lymph nodes. It is believed that the fungal *antigens*, a substance that causes your body to produce antibodies, leaked from the lymph nodes and into the mediastinal space causing a hypersensitive reaction and resulted in an "exuberant fibrotic response." [xvi] that cause a build-up of calcium salts that harden into *calcifications*. These invasive calcifications cause obstruction by pressing against or wrapping around vessels, airways and organs. Obstructions cause blockage of blood flow between the heart, lungs and the rest of the body by wrapping around pulmonary arteries and vena cavae. They can also obstruct the trachea and other airways, inhibiting the ability of air to get into the lungs. Some patients have esophageal involvement that makes it difficult or impossible for them to swallow. It is not until these obstructions occur that most people with FM are diagnosed. [xvii]

According to Dr. Loyd, "Most patients probably were initially infected with Histoplasmosis in their youth. It appears that the scar process grows at about one millimeter per year, so it is very slow-growing and it may take several years before it leads to obstruction of the large arteries, veins or airways."[xviii]

The reason for this dramatic reaction in some hosts is also not understood, although researchers are looking into genetic influences, such as those with the *HLA-A2 antigen.* [xix] (Those self-made antigens that are supposed to protect you from yourself.) The complexities of human leukocyte antigen serotypes go way beyond the scope of this book.

In the end we are left with random calcified masses that surgeons have described as a woody substance. It is nearly impossible to remove surgically and is, therefore, almost never a treatment option.

When it was first described to me I was told it was as if someone has poured molten plastic over my organs and let it harden. Other surgeons describe the fibrosis as "concrete" that encases structures. This makes it unwise to do any type of surgical intervention and even makes it impossible to perform a transplant.

Fibrosing mediastinitis has been described as insidious and progressive, although physicians disagree as to the rate or type of progression.

Race, age, and sex do not seem to be factors, but statistics vary slightly. In independent surveys, the average patient has been a Caucasian female diagnosed during her late 30's to early 40's. In a study from 1986 that involved 94 patients, the average age was 33 years (range, 1 to 83 years.) For every female there were one and half males and eighty-one percent of the patients were white. [xx] In the Vanderbilt studies, the mean age of diagnosis was 37 years. Sixty-six percent of patients were women and 74% were Caucasian.

How We Become Derailed

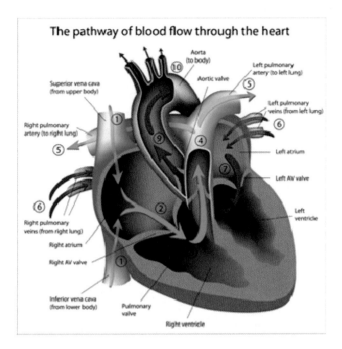

The pathway of blood flow through the heart

Structures of the mediastinum include the heart and its vessels. These vessels are common structures to be affected by fibrosing mediastinitis. The occlusion of vessels, such as the pulmonary arteries, pulmonary veins, and vena cavae is a primary reason why FM can be so devastating.

The heart is a pump whose primary purpose is to deliver oxygen-rich blood (red blood) to the tissues of the body. The heart and lungs are intimately connected, working as a team to transport oxygen into the cells. The lungs bring oxygen into the body, but must rely on the heart to help deliver it to the rest of the body. This works in a constant cycle, with every beat of our hearts.

The heart is made up of specialized muscle tissue not found anywhere else in the body. The heart has four chambers: two upper chambers called *atria* (singular: atrium) and two lower chambers called *ventricles*.

Electrical impulses cause the specialized heart muscle to contract (systole) and rest (diastole) in order to move blood from chamber to chamber and into the rest of the body. The brief rest period gives the heart chambers a chance to fill with blood while the contraction forces the blood into the lungs and the other body tissues. Blood returns to the heart through veins and leaves the heart through arteries.

When red blood cells are depleted of their oxygen they return to the heart through large veins called the *vena cavae*. The vena cavae delivers the blood into the right atrium. Blood from the upper body (head, neck, arms) returns through the superior vena cava (SVC), while the blood from the lower body returns via the inferior vena cava (IVC). When the right atrium is filled with blood it opens a valve (tricuspid) and the blood passively enters the right ventricle. The contraction of the heart muscle then squeezes the blood from the right ventricle into the lungs by way of the main pulmonary artery. The main pulmonary artery divides into a right and left pulmonary artery that go to the right and left lung respectively.

The oxygen exchange occurs in the lungs' air sacs, known as *alveoli* and the oxygen-rich blood is dumped back into the heart, this time into the left atrium. Once the left atrium is filled, the valve between the left atrium and the left ventricle, the mitral valve, opens, allowing the blood to enter the left ventricle. When the heart contracts it forces the blood into the rest of the body through a large artery called the aorta. The oxygen is delivered to the tissues and the whole cycle begins again. Normally, there will be 70-90 cycles occurring every minute.

I like to think of red blood cells as train cars delivering little boxes of oxygen molecules. The veins and arteries are the rail system. The lungs are the supplier and the cells of the body are the awaiting consumers. In a healthy human, this system works well. The train track is always clear, the cargo is always available and the cells are happy customers.

What happens when the train system is blocked? This is precisely what happens in many cases of fibrosing mediastinitis. The track is blocked somewhere and the train cannot pick up cargo or deliver it to the consumer.

For example, if the superior vena cava is blocked, then the empty train cars get backed up. This is known as *superior vena cava syndrome*. (SVC syndrome) It can be the result of other disease processes, but is one of the most common problems caused by FM. Blood can't adequately return to the heart from the head, neck and upper extremities to pick up oxygen from the lungs. The train cars back up and cause a massive congestion. People with SVC syndrome experience extreme discomfort due to swelling of the face, neck, and arms. This swelling can also compress other structures and lead to difficulty breathing or eating. The body tries to alleviate this traffic jam by creating new vessels called *collaterals*. This is merely a network of detours that develop in the body's desperate attempt to relieve the pressure. Sometimes collaterals will be enough to alleviate the symptoms, but in many cases intervention is necessary.

In other cases, the FM can block one or both pulmonary arteries or veins. For instance, if the left pulmonary artery is blocked by FM, the empty train cars can't get to the supplier to pick up their cargo. They get diverted to the right pulmonary artery and try to pick up cargo from the right lung. Now the right lung is trying to supply twice as many train cars and it becomes overwhelmed. The demand exceeds the supply and the system goes haywire. The body tries to make do with one supplier, but it's not always easy.

People with pulmonary artery blockages from FM experience symptoms such as shortness of breath, chest pain, hemoptysis (coughing up blood), and fatigue. They experience many of the same symptoms as a person who has a *pulmonary embolism* or *PE*.

In some cases, if both pulmonary arteries are partially or completely blocked a person's health will be extremely compromised and their prognosis is usually poor. The small supply of oxygen cannot meet the demands of the tissues.

Superior Vena Cava (SVC) Syndrome is the most common manifestation of fibrosing mediastinitis. Patients will typically seek treatment when they notice facial, arm and/or neck swelling. They may be misdiagnosed with such things ranging from a pinched nerve to a thyroid disorder before a diagnosis of FM.

Pulmonary artery obstruction is also common, but a majority (Vanderbilt estimated 80%) of patients only have one lung involved, most commonly the right. There is some disagreement about whether or not intervention is worthwhile in patients with only one lung involved. It is believed that people with one functioning lung are able to live relatively normal lives.

(I know patients who would disagree with this.) If multiple vessels are involved in one lung, then treatment becomes even more difficult.

Chronic *pleuritic* chest pain is common in people with pulmonary vascular occlusion and will vary in intensity for every person. Some people can manage with anti-inflammatory medications while others need narcotic pain relief.

Hemoptysis is also common due to growth of arteries in the affected lung. Occasionally, a procedure must be done to embolize (cut off or clamp) the bleeding areas.

If a person has one lung involved it is not likely that his/her FM will spread to the opposite lung. "Post-Histo FM rarely, if ever, extends to new sites where there was not mediastinal proliferation at the time of the initial diagnosis."[xxi] However, the prognosis for individuals with bilateral involvement is usually grim. These folks usually have vascular and airway invasion as well. The combination of right pulmonary artery followed later by left mainstem bronchial obstruction is the most common manifestation.

Treatment Options for Vascular Invasion

The treatments for vascular obstruction are varied. Some patients with SVC syndrome may not need any intervention since they can develop collateral circulation that relieves their symptoms. Others undergo surgical intervention to have a bypass with a spiral vein graft harvested from a large vein in the leg (saphenous) or an artificial graft to alleviate the *stenosis* (narrowing).

Over the last 10 years, the use of endovascular stenting has become more widespread. Clinicians are less inclined to stent an SVC in patients who do not exhibit complications of SVC syndrome. Also, it has been found that these patients develop collateral circulation enough to compensate for the dysfunction of the SVC.

Pulmonary artery obstruction due to FM has been treated both surgically and with stenting. The Texas Heart Institute performed a successful bypass in a patient with bilateral pulmonary artery involvement. [xxii] Some physicians feel that surgical bypass is preferable over stenting, as stents may only relieve symptoms for a short period of time. Again, the challenges of surgical intervention come into play due to the nature of the fibrosis.

One of the biggest problems with receiving treatment for vascular obstruction due to FM is finding a skilled clinician who is willing and/or able to perform the necessary procedure. Although cardiac catheterizations are routinely done on patients in many facilities across the United States and in the world, they are not sufficient when dealing with patients with FM. Routine cardiac catheterizations for cardiac patients do not involve passing a catheter through chambers of the heart. Catheterizations for FM patients, whose vena cavae and pulmonary arteries and veins are affected, are more invasive. These procedures also may require a patient to undergo general anesthesia, a risk in and of itself.

There are certainly risks to pulmonary vascular stenting and it would be up to you and your specialist to decide if these risks make it infeasible. Studies at Vanderbilt have shown that about 25% of patients make it to the cath lab only to discover that they cannot be stented. There have been reports of aortic laceration after SVC stenting. Other complications include pulmonary artery dissection, reperfusion pulmonary edema, pulmonary hemorrhage, hypoxia requiring supplemental oxygen for several weeks, cerebral vascular accident (stroke), and in-stent *thrombosis.* [xxiii]

The criteria for stenting are somewhat rigid. Some patients who have had stenting for FM have typically received treatment from pediatric interventionalists as they have more experience with pulmonary arteries. Some physicians believe that stenting is not an option for people with only one vessel involved.

There is one reported instance of carotid artery stenosis from fibrosing mediastinitis. A 54-year-old woman began experiencing neurologic symptoms from extension of a known mediastinal mass resulting in 70% to 79% stenosis of the right internal carotid artery. The stenosis was treated with endovascular stenting. Completion angiogram revealed a good result with <10% residual stenosis. At 18-month follow-up, the patient was symptom free without evidence of re-stenosis. [xxiv]

Pulmonary Hypertension

When pulmonary vasculature is compromised it is possible to develop a secondary condition called pulmonary hypertension. Pulmonary hypertension is abnormally high blood pressure in the arteries of the lungs. It makes the right side of the heart work harder than normal.

Blood from the body enters the right side of the heart where it is pumped into the lungs to pick up oxygen. Then the oxygenated blood is returned to the left side of the heart where it is then pumped out to the rest of the body.

When arteries in the lungs become occluded or narrow, the blood cannot adequately move between the heart and the lungs. The pressure caused from this is called pulmonary hypertension. The heart must work harder to push against the narrowed vessels and, as a result, the right side of the heart becomes larger.

Have you ever taken a child's balloon and blown it up to its maximum capacity and let the air out? If you do this over and over again have you noticed how the balloon becomes weak and boggy? That's what happens to the heart with pulmonary hypertension. When the right side of the heart fails it is called *cor pulmonale.*

When pulmonary hypertension has a known cause, it is called secondary pulmonary hypertension. Some causes of pulmonary hypertension include:

- Autoimmune diseases that damage the lungs, such as scleroderma and rheumatoid arthritis

- Birth defects of the heart

- Pulmonary embolism

- Congestive heart failure

- Heart valve disease

- HIV

- Chronic low levels of oxygen in the blood
- Certain medications (Fen-Phen and other appetite suppressants have been linked to pulmonary hypertension)

- Recreational drugs such as methamphetamine and cocaine

- Low oxygen levels in the blood for a long time (chronic)

- Lung disease, such as COPD or pulmonary fibrosis

- Obstructive sleep apnea

Sometimes the cause is unknown. Remember that term idiopathic? Idiopathic pulmonary arterial hypertension or IPAH, has no known definite cause. It also affects more women than men.

Shortness of breath or light-headedness during activity is often the first symptom. A person may also experience palpitations, but this is not helpful to people who have FM since 90% of them experience these symptoms regularly. Gradually, these symptoms worsen and occur even at rest. Other symptoms include:

- Lower extremity swelling

- Cyanosis (turning blue)

- Chest pain or pressure, usually in the front of the chest

- Dizziness or fainting spells

- Fatigue

- Increased belly size

- Weakness

On examination, a physician may notice an abnormal heart sound or murmur, distended neck veins, a pulsation over the sternum, and/or lower extremity edema.

Tests used to diagnose pulmonary hypertension include lab tests, chest CT, cardiac catheterization (directly measures the pressures in the vessels), and echocardiogram. There are other tests that may be useful such as EKG, x-rays, nuclear scans, sleep studies and an exercise tolerance test called a six minute walk test.

There is no known cure for pulmonary hypertension. Treatment goals include control of symptoms and to treat the underlying cause.

Some forms of pulmonary hypertension are treated with medications such as Ambrisentan (Letairis), Bosentan (Tracleer), Calcium channel blockers, diuretics, Prostacyclin or similar medicines, and sildenafil.(yes, Viagra). Physicians may also prescribe a blood thinner to keep blood clots from forming.

Let's Take a Deep Breath

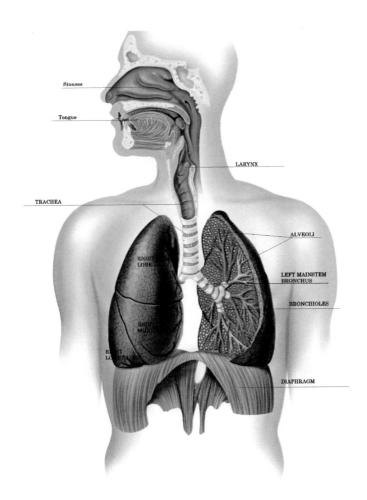

When we take a breath, air passes through our nose and mouth through our voice box (*larynx*) and into our trachea or windpipe. The trachea is a rigid structure made up of rings of cartilage. The trachea then branches into two main *bronchi* (singular *bronchus*) that enter the right and left lung. The junction where they divide is called the *carina*. Each bronchus then divides into various *bronchioles* inside the lungs and terminates into the lung tissue's *alveoli* where oxygen is exchanged with the bloodstream.

The *diaphragm* is the main muscle used in breathing. It is a dome-shaped muscle at the bottom of the lungs that separates the chest cavity from the abdominal cavity. (It is also what spasms when you have hiccups). When the diaphragm contracts, it flattens out and causes the space where the lungs lie to expand, which draws air into the lungs. When the diaphragm expands, the chest cavity is reduced and air is pushed out of the lungs.

There are two lungs, right and left. The right lung is made up of three sections called *lobes*. The left lung only has two lobes. The lungs are made up of about 700 million alveoli so the lungs, when out of the body, feel like a cushy sponge and not solid as you might expect. The lungs and thoracic cavity are lined with a thin membrane called pleura. There is an inner, or visceral, pleural membrane around the lungs and an outer, or parietal, pleural membrane lining the inside of the rib cage and the diaphragm. The space between the two layers is called the pleural space. Sometimes this space can fill with fluid and cause a pleural effusion. The inflammation of the pleural membranes is called *pleurisy or pleuritis.*

A *thoracotomy* is the process of making an incision into the chest wall. The surgical removal of your lung is called a *pneumonectomy.* If they only take out a lobe then it is called a *lobectomy.*

Other complications of fibrosing mediastinitis, although less common, include airway compression that can lead to pneumonia or collapse of the lung (*atelectasis*). All those little air sacs collapse, preventing the exchange of oxygen. Calcified lymph nodes can also cause bronchial erosion, which can cause bleeding. Patients may also develop inflammation of the bronchi caused by an accumulation of hard concretions or stones on their lining called broncholithiasis.[xxv] Bronchial obstruction seems to occur more on the left side than on the right. These patients typically have symptoms of wheezing, coughing, or chronic respiratory tract infections. [xxvi]

Interventions for Airway Complications

The treatment of airway obstruction is challenging. Sometimes the fibrotic mass is so dense and the airway is so rigid that dilation is impossible. Whereas stents may be used to open blood vessels and restore blood flow, the same is not true for airways. Airway stents, known as tracheobronchial prostheses, are varied. The main classes of stents are silicone, metal, and hybrid.

Silicone stents are the most common. They are firm, stable in high temperatures and well tolerated. They resist compression from external problems such as tumors or enlarged lymph nodes. Once this type of stent is placed it can generally be repositioned easily, which also makes it easier to dislodge or migrate accidentally.

Metal stents have a few advantages. They can be inserted under bronchoscopy with procedural sedation. They rarely migrate and self-expanding metal stents may distend firm strictures. This is especially beneficial when an airway cannot be dilated beforehand. One disadvantage is the greater risk of airway perforation. They are also difficult, if not impossible to remove. Granulation tissue easily grows through the spaces of uncovered metal stents that may lead to obstruction.[xxvii]

Hybrid stents are made of two or more material and are designed to overcome the issues related to metal and silicone stents. They may employ the strength of metal but the protection of the silicone.

If a lesion causing airway stenosis cannot be resected (surgically removed), then experts believe that dilation is necessary before stent placement. Fibrosing mediastinitis is, by nature, one of the most impossible lesions to resect. Surgery is possible, but technically difficult and has an undesirable mortality rate. [xxviii] In the cases where *resection* is impossible, the use of sequential stents of increasing size can be inserted. This is usually done with silicone stents since they are easier to remove.

Stents can be effective, but there is often need for reintervention. The removal of stents can be very difficult, especially with metal stents. Studies show that 58 percent of procedures to remove a metal stent resulted in a complication, most commonly re-obstruction, followed by respiratory failure.[xxix]

Complications of stents are typically not life-threatening. The insertion of stents can cause an inflammatory reaction and result in granulation tissue forming on the ends of the stents. Obstruction of the stent by secretions or regrowth of a lesion may occur. The stent can migrate (move) with coughing or lesion growth. Airway wall perforation, stent rupture, broken wires or metal fatigue are all potential complications. [xxx]

Chronic infections due to airway obstruction have been treated with surgeries such as removal of the entire lung (*pneumonectomy*). Obviously, this may complicate a person's life by diminishing their respiratory capacity even more.

Esophageal Complications

People who have fibrosing mediastinitis may also have compression or narrowing of the esophagus, the tube that runs from the mouth to the stomach. Typically, these people will have symptoms of difficulty swallowing (*dysphagia*), chest pain, and/or pain with swallowing (*odynophagia*).

Esophageal involvement is not one of the most common complications with fibrosing mediastinitis. This could be due to the thick walls of the esophagus, its distensibility, and motility or it could be that the fibrosis usually spares the posterior mediastinum. [xxxi]

It is possible for fibrosing mediastinitis to cause a traction diverticulum, a localized distortion, angulation, or funnel-shaped bulging of the esophageal wall, due to adhesions resulting from an external lesion. Mild cases do not need treatment. Others that cause difficulty swallowing can be remedied with dilation of the esophagus.

Esophageal dilatation is the most common treatment, although there have been rare instances when a patient must undergo an esophagectomy, removing part or the entire esophagus. The esophagus is then reconstructed using part of the stomach.

The trachea and esophagus lie very close to one another within the mediastinum. A serious complication that could arise is a *tracheobronchoesophageal fistula* (TEF) where the walls of the esophagus erode through and connect to the trachea or bronchus. This results in air going where the food should go and food going where the air should go. Neither is good. This requires immediate surgery. The bronchoesophogeal fistulas most commonly occur in the subcarinal (below the junction of the trachea) space between the esophagus and the right mainstem bronchus. [xxxii]

Gastro-esophageal reflux is a common problem in the general population, but is probably not directly related to FM.

Pharmaceutical Treatment

There are no drugs that have shown to be effective against fibrosing mediastinitis. Some clinicians will prescribe itraconazole, an antifungal in order to treat what may be left of the Histoplasmosis, but it is often the case that FM patients are way past the infection of Histo and the use of antifungals is not helpful.

The use of corticosteroids such as Prednisone is also controversial. Some physicians believe it may diminish inflammation and is, in some cases, useful in acute flare-ups, but overall it is not effective against fibrosing mediastinitis.

Some patients are on blood thinners such as Coumadin (warfarin). Coumadin keeps the blood from forming clots and must be regulated carefully. Your doctor will do a blood test routinely to check your *prothrombin time INR* or PT/INR. The INR must stay within a therapeutic range (typically 2.0-2.5). The greatest risk of Coumadin is uncontrolled bleeding.

People with Fibrosing Mediastinitis

I am grateful to the people who have graciously agreed to be part of this book. Some of them live fairly normal lives, while others face daily challenges of pain and uncertainty.

I came in contact with most of these people through the Facebook group or through my website, seeking information about their disease. I consider it a privilege to tell their stories.

As you will see, many of them were misdiagnosed for years before they were told they had fibrosing mediastinitis. Even with a diagnosis, things did not become easier because the condition is rare and there are very few medical professionals who understand or treat it.

Their stories are told from their own perspectives. I have merely edited their stories and have attempted to explain the clinical aspects of what they have reported to me. I have not seen anyone's medical records nor do I try to offer an explanation for their symptoms. Some of them have other illnesses that may or may not be directly related to their FM. It should not be concluded that diseases, such as gastrointestinal disease, diabetes, liver disease or other cardiac or respiratory diseases are brought on by fibrosing mediastinitis. There has been very little studied about the correlation of FM and other conditions. There are, however, schools of thought that are considering that other autoimmune diseases may occur in patients with FM, but studies are, at this time, inconclusive.

Many of the people that contributed to DERAILED expressed similar concerns. They feel that their disease is misunderstood by, not only the medical community, but by their families and friends. There are no obvious outward signs that someone has FM, unless they're on oxygen. Therefore, FM can be a "hidden disability." Many tell me, "I look pretty good on the outside, but I feel bad on the inside." Most of them live with chronic chest pain, shortness of breath, and fatigue, often to the point where they are no longer able to work. Some have received interventions that have allowed them to return to a fairly normal life while others have been told their condition is beyond treatment.

The people in DERAILED will tell you how FM affects their lives, relationships, job, and sense of self. They share fears and frustrations. They have fear of the unknown about how their lives will change, and in some cases, end. They express frustrations about the lack of information and medical resources for their condition. Many don't understand what is happening inside their bodies. Some express anger that they were misdiagnosed or about the possibility that their condition could have been prevented. "My doctor doesn't know anything about my disease," some say. "I don't know where to go to get help."

The following section contains many medical terms. Words with italics are described in the glossary at the end of the book.

Tami

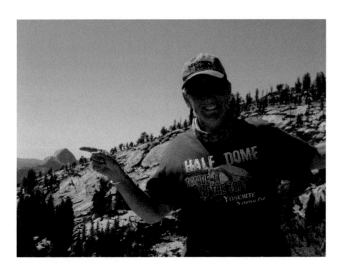

I was born in New Jersey, but was raised in the Ohio Valley. My childhood was spent playing in the woods around our home. I had the usual run of childhood illnesses, but nothing very serious, except for a bout of scarlet fever when I was six.

I graduated from nursing school in 1986 and worked in intensive care and the emergency department. During the mid-1990's I had what seemed to be a never-ending respiratory infection. My family doctor would put me on antibiotics, but I never seemed to get over it. I persuaded him to let me go and see a pulmonologist.

As soon as the pulmonologist saw me he told me I had asthma. He put me on inhalers and I accepted my fate. I continued to have a frequent cough and shortness of breath, but I just accepted that this was normal.

One day, while I was at work, taking care of a patient in the recovery room, I completely lost my vision. Everything went dark. I had no other symptoms, but I was alarmed. One of my co-workers took me across the street to the eye center where I sat in the waiting room, blind, for nearly an hour. During that time, my vision gradually came back. The doctor finally examined me and declared that I had an "ocular migraine." The same thing happened during the summer of 1999 while I was cleaning my apartment. It lasted a bit longer, but I attributed to this "ocular migraine" and didn't worry about it as much.

Over the Labor Day weekend in 1999, I began having terrible chest pain. Every breath felt like a knife going through my chest. I went to the ER to be evaluated. Chest x-rays, blood gases, and blood work turned up nothing, but the doctor taking care of me that day, Dr. Michael Bain, was insistent that my symptoms were not normal. He didn't like the fact that my resting heart rate was over 110.

Because I had recently returned from a long road trip, he ordered a lung scan to see whether I had a pulmonary embolism. The lung scan showed complete occlusion of my left pulmonary artery; that is, I was getting no blood flow to my left lung. I thought I had a pulmonary embolism, but I was told that the cause of my obstruction was, most likely, a mass. It would be impossible to biopsy the mass because it was lying against the artery. The radiologist believed a blood clot had formed inside the vessel. A needle biopsy would certainly result in severe bleeding. I was hospitalized and placed on blood thinners. The obstruction in my artery was also, most likely, the cause of my earlier temporary blindness.

Next, I was taken for a pulmonary angiogram to evaluate whether or not I had a blood clot. Then I had a *bronchoscopy* to evaluate whether or not I had cancer cells in my lungs. I was sedated, but I remember the scope going into my nose and straight down into my lungs which caused severe coughing and discomfort.

I spent the next several days in the hospital, growing more short of breath and having more pain than I had previously. At one point I got into the shower and was unable to get back to bed without help. They told me that my life would be like this because I was living with one lung, but no one had explained what was happening to me. I could not understand how I'd gotten so much worse in just a few days. The doctors told me they would re-evaluate me in a few months. I was sent home with pain pills and blood thinners, but no real diagnosis.

The night I got home I was awakened in the middle of the night with severe pain and shortness of breath. I called my brother who took me immediately back to the hospital where I ended up in the ICU on blood thinners and morphine for the severe pain. I was in and out of awareness because of the drugs and a few times I thought my life was really over. My mom stayed with me most of the time.

I knew most of the nurses who were taking care of me since I worked with them. They were extremely attentive and protective and I had visitors all the time. At one point, a close friend I knew from college showed up from Columbus. It was atypical of her to wander far from home so when I saw her standing in my doorway I felt a sense of dread. "Oh, geez, I must be dying," I told her. We still laugh about that.

Several doctors consulted on my case. I was taken to the radiology department where they placed a *PICC line* in my left arm. The thoracic surgeon felt the best thing to do would be to take out my lung, a treatment I was not too keen about. I refused to have it done. No one seemed to know what to do with me. There was discussion of sending me to either Vanderbilt in Tennessee, Mayo Clinic in Minnesota or to UCSD in San Diego.

Three days later, I ended up on a plane bound for Cleveland Clinic. A parade of my friends and co-workers lined the hallway from the ICU through the ER and out to the awaiting ambulance. Later, I found out that one of the nurses told my close friend, "She's not coming back." I was never fully aware of how sick I was.

My mom boarded the tiny plane with me. I don't remember anything about the flight as they had sedated me with Ativan and morphine. An ambulance transported me from the airport to Cleveland Clinic where I was initially placed on a medical unit.

The flight nurse said, "I will not leave this patient here. I took her out of ICU and I'll take her right back."

I was in and out of coherence because of the morphine, but I remember thinking, *My god, they're going to put me back on the plane and take me home.*

Somehow I ended up in a monitored step-down unit. All of the special care I'd received at my home hospital was gone. I called my doctor back home and begged him to let me go back to Cincinnati. I was scared. He told me I was exactly where I needed to be. My begging was futile. I was stuck.

I had no idea what was going to happen to me. I had strange dreams. I woke up when I thought I was already awake. I would hear people in my room that weren't there and on more than one occasion I felt someone tapping on the bottom of my feet. I thought it was my mom, but each time I opened my eyes to see her there was no one in the room. I was scared, but tried to keep my sense of humor. I thought about all the things I hadn't done in my life.

I was taken to the cardiac cath lab where I underwent a rather unpleasant catheterization. The doctor went through my jugular vein as opposed to the femoral I had previously had accessed. The radiologist was rough and was aggravated that the catheter would not go into the space he wanted. I was forced to keep my head turned to the left and they had placed this strange wooden box that covered my face.

As a critical care nurse, I had helped with several of these procedures. I knew that passing a catheter through the heart could cause irregular heartbeats or dysrhythmias. It was even possible to put a patient into a fatal arrhythmia. I could feel my heart palpitating when the doctor attempted to place the catheter through my heart, causing these dysrhythmias. The nurse counted off the abnormal beats and I tried to concentrate on what was going on, thinking to myself: *As long as I can hear her voice, I'm alright.*

Finally, I was taken back to my room. The sheath was left in my neck and stuck out past my right ear. I could feel it stabbing every time I moved my head. The catheter tip was in my pulmonary artery near the blockage and the clot.

The plan was to instill a continuous infusion of *tPa*, a clot-busting enzymatic drug. The drug also caused severe bleeding because it inhibited natural clotting in the body. The infusion would last for several hours throughout the night.

During the night the PICC site and the catheter in my neck bled continuously. The urine in my catheter was crimson. Blood ran down my neck to my chest and onto the bed. Blood spurted out from the PICC site every time I moved my arm. The nurse placed pads underneath my arm to catch the blood and took away heavily saturated pads all during the night.

"Quit moving your arm," she scolded me. She wanted me to hold my arm in an unnatural position to keep the blood from coming out. The whole thing was a nightmare. I was worried about losing so much blood, but no one seemed to be too concerned.

In the morning a resident I'd never seen came in and said, "Oh, you're bleeding too much." *That's what I'd been thinking.* They stopped the tPA infusion and I was taken back to the cardiac cath lab where they checked the status of the occlusion. Nothing had changed. The radiologist said very little to me. He yanked the catheter from my neck and walked out, leaving me on the table. On his way out he said, "Your lymph nodes are all enlarged." I had no idea what that meant and no one explained to us what was going on. I was taken back to my room.

The next procedure they wanted to do was a mediastinoscopy, a surgery where they would make an incision in my neck, put a scope into my chest and biopsy the mass. I waited around for several days while the tPA got out of my system, but I remained on a Heparin drip. The surgeon came in and explained the procedure and told me the Heparin drip would be turned off the night before my surgery.

Around 2am on the night before my surgery, I noticed my Heparin drip was still going. I called the nurse in and told her what the surgeon had said. "We don't have an order to turn it off," she informed me.

"Well, you better get an order because I'm not waiting around another day to have this surgery."

I was frustrated because I'd waited for three days as it was and I still did not know what was wrong with me. I had very little confidence in Cleveland Clinic at this point. A short time later, the Heparin was turned off.

The next day I was taken to the huge surgical suite where two doctors spoke to me in a French accent. One took my right hand and plunged a needle into my radial artery to start an arterial line. The next thing I remember is that I was waking up in the recovery unit, my throat very sore and hoarse. I now had a suture line across my throat. The next day I was up and about and feeling a little better, but I still had the pain and was pretty weak.

My mom and I spent a lot of time sitting outside by the fountain and walking through the hospital.

Another pulmonary resident, a frumpy woman with whitish hair who I had never seen before, came in to see me. She said something about "your diagnosis."

My mom said, "What *is* her diagnosis?"

The resident looked at us. "You mean you don't know?"

"No," we said in unison. "No one's told us anything."

"You have fibrosing mediastinitis."

I'd been a nurse for several years and my mom had worked in the medical field even longer and neither of us had ever heard these words before.

"What do we do about it?" my mom asked.

"There's nothing to do about it. There's no cure and it's progressive. I'm sorry." Then she told us that it was caused from a Histoplasmosis infection. I never had asthma. We were stunned. I had a disease we'd never heard of and I was most likely going to die from it.

Finally, after a few more days, they weaned me from the blood thinners and started me on Coumadin. I was taking Sporanox, an anti-fungal drug, and Prednisone. I was released from Cleveland Clinic.

A family friend flew me home in his private plane. I returned to my apartment, but did not return to work for several weeks. I went to the hospital for a routine blood test about a week after I returned home to check if my blood was thin enough with the Coumadin. I ran into the thoracic surgeon that had taken care of me before I was sent to Cleveland. He asked me why my voice was hoarse. I could barely speak above a whisper, but I had attributed it to the endotracheal tube that had been placed during my surgery.

He said, "Your voice should be normal now. I think you should have it checked out."

I made an appointment with an ENT specialist. He put a scope into my nose and down my throat to evaluate my vocal cords. He told me they were paralyzed. He didn't know if my voice would come back so he gave me two options: I could wait to see if my voice would come back on its own or I could have him remove and repair my larynx.

Having already had my neck probed and slashed within the past three weeks, I wasn't too motivated to have more surgery. I opted to wait. I called the surgeon in Cleveland Clinic who had performed my mediastinoscopy and he said, "Yes, I probably knocked your laryngeal nerve around. Let me know if your voice isn't back by spring." This was October.

I returned to Cleveland Clinic to follow-up with the pulmonologist. He told us that I was still having chest pain because I was "throwing clots" to my lung. He told me that they could not stent my pulmonary artery because it was so narrow they could hardly get a guide wire into the opening. There was no surgery that would help. His only advice was to "live my life." He could not give me a prognosis; only telling me that people with my disease live until their early 40's. He told me to seek help if I had more pain, more shortness of breath or started coughing up blood.

Back home, I persuaded my supervisor to let me return to work even though I was still short of breath and had no voice. I also still had a pleuritic pain. She told me that I should consider going on disability, but I told her there may be a time when I really would have to go on disability and I wanted to wait. She allowed me to return to 4-hour shifts, then 8 hours and gradually back to 12 hours. I couldn't speak very loudly which made it difficult to talk to hard-of-hearing patients. My co-workers gave me a whistle to use in case I needed help because I could not yell.

By mid-November my voice started to return on its own. I had always wanted to travel so I started looking into travel nurse jobs. I was a little scared about leaving my job, but I was feeling fairly well and thought I should seize the opportunity. I also had an ulterior motive.

Against the advice of my friends, I decided to take a job in San Diego, California. My thought was that if I ever got sicker I'd be close to University of California San Diego (UCSD). I moved myself to San Diego and did pretty well for a while.

A couple of months later, I began to have episodes where my feet and hands would turn blue. I was often short of breath and my endurance level was very low. I had been having chest pain every day since the previous summer and I was learning to live with it, but in the spring of 2000, it had gotten worse. I had more severe pain and a co-worker who worked part-time in the ER at UCSD took me to Thornton Hospital in La Jolla. I was admitted under the care of a pulmonologist named Dr. Kim Kerr.

I had developed a pericardial and pleural effusion that caused severe pain. Dr. Kerr would stand outside the door of my room where she could actually hear my lung squeaking as I breathed. "That hurts, doesn't it?" she asked.

She gave me a dose of Solu-Medrol which dramatically reduced my pain. She reviewed my history and ordered an MRI which showed that I probably never had a blood clot, but that the fibrosis had completely encased my pulmonary artery.

She said to me, "I have a friend who is a pediatric cardiologist. He has tiny instruments and I think he can do an angiogram on you." She knew I had been told that my artery could not be stented so she made no promises. I was taken, by ambulance, from Thornton Hospital to the main hospital in Hillcrest in downtown San Diego.

On May 9, 2000, I underwent another pulmonary angiogram with Dr. Abraham Rothman. This time I was asleep for the four hour long procedure. When I awakened the first thing I was told was that Dr. Rothman managed to open my pulmonary artery with 2 stents. I was taken to the ICU where I spent the night in case I went into flash pulmonary edema, a possible side effect of having a sudden rush of blood to my lung that had not had circulation for a long time.

Fortunately, I suffered no ill effects. Dr. Kerr had another lung scan done the next day and the blood flow to my lung seemed to have disappeared. Once again, I went back to the cath lab to have the stents checked. The angiogram showed that everything was working fine.

I was released from the hospital on Coumadin and a few days later I was in my truck driving back to Ohio. The experience at UCSD was the antithesis of my grim hospitalization at Cleveland Clinic.

For a few years I did really well. In 2002, I met my partner, Monica, and settled on the central California coast. The pulmonologist I went to on the central coast told me outright, "I don't want to be your doctor. I don't know anything about your disease." He encouraged me to go back to San Diego.

I had episodes of chest pain that sometimes became more severe, but tests always showed that my blood flow was adequate. Usually, I would be placed on short-term steroid treatment and the pain would subside to its usual tolerable level.

Living with this disease is still frightening and frustrating at times. In December of 2002 I returned to San Diego to see Dr. Kerr in hopes that she could shed light on why I was still having chest pain. She told me I could have another MRI, but, she warned, if the mass was changing there was nothing she could do about it.

She did an echocardiogram to make sure I wasn't developing pulmonary hypertension. It was normal. She told me I would have "flare-ups" and that they should be treated with steroids. I opted not to have the MRI because I only wanted to concentrate on things I could have fixed.

Over the next few years I noticed my stamina decreasing and my flare-ups becoming more frequent. I visited another pulmonologist who told me that I needed to have another angiogram to check my stents. I knew it was the prudent thing to do, but the truth was that no one in my insurance network was willing or able to do a pulmonary angiogram, and if they did, they would not be able to do any interventions.

Nearly a year went by until summer 2006 when I developed some of the worst pain I had ever had. I thought it was just another flare-up, but something told me it was more serious. I was also experiencing more fatigue and having blackout spells when I'd lift or stretch. I tried to wait it out, but I ended up going to the ER where, once again, I was told I needed to have an angiogram to check the stents. I realized the best thing to do was to try to find Dr. Rothman and ask him what to do.

A few days later I found Dr. Rothman after searching for him on the Internet. He told me he wanted to do the angiogram himself and wanted me to make arrangements to fly to Las Vegas where he was now practicing.

In September 2006, Monica and I flew to Las Vegas and met up with my mom who flew from Ohio. Dr. Rothman examined me and was not surprised by any of my symptoms. The angiogram revealed that my stents had nearly closed off completely. He said I was as ill as I had been when he first met me in San Diego. Apparently, the tissue in my vessels grew through the stent and closed them off.

"You're a tissue grower," Dr. Rothman told me.

Amazingly, using balloon angioplasty, he managed to open the stents up even more than he had initially six years before. The next day, I could tell the difference in how I felt.

I followed up with Dr. Rothman in March 2009 and had another angioplasty. This time my artery was not as closed and he felt it would be possible for me to wait longer before doing another procedure.

As far as I know, my FM has not spread. I still have chest pain periodically with shortness of breath. Two times I have received narcotic pain killers for unrelated conditions and developed the worst pain of my life. I am not entirely clear what that is all about, but I think it may be related to my FM and the low perfusion of blood to my chest. I don't tolerate high altitudes well, but I basically live a normal life. I no longer take my health for granted. Living with FM has opened my eyes to what is important: love, family, and experiencing as much as you can.

Tricia

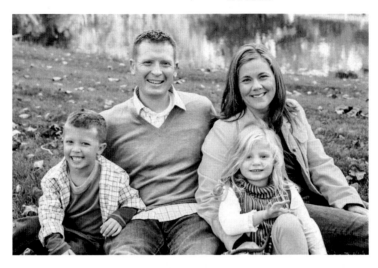

Fibrosing Mediastinitis: Two words that I had never heard before, but have become a part of my everyday language. I've learned to spell it and say it so when it falls on the ears of someone who also has never heard it, I hopefully only have to say it once.

It was life changing, certainly, but I am at the point where I can reflect back and I can't imagine my life without it. I am blessed that the disease seems to have stabilized and my quality of life has been great.

It wasn't always that way, and if not for the intervention that Dr. Loyd and Dr. Doyle (Vanderbilt Medical Center) were able to perform on my SVC, my life would most likely have ended several years ago, a thought that humbles me often.

I grew up in Grand Ledge, Michigan, just outside of the Lansing city limits. We rarely traveled during my childhood. Sadly, my father had multiple sclerosis and his progression with the disease was ongoing, spanning over my entire childhood. I did see, firsthand, a disease that cripples and steals the quality of life that I am so grateful for. I've realized that I will never know where I contracted histoplasmosis and I've accepted that fact. It does cross my mind for my children occasionally. Although I am quickly rooted and realize if I were to try and protect them from life's unseen dangers, they'd have to live in a bubble.

I am grateful for my quick diagnosis, another realization that, in hindsight, became clear. After hearing many stories of fellow FM survivors, my path to an accurate diagnosis was swift.

My symptoms started during the summer of my 32nd year. I was single at the time and enjoyed working out, gardening, and travel. It was after a run on a Sunday afternoon when I was stretching and I felt an incredible fullness in my neck. The sensation was exactly what it felt like when I was a child hanging upside down on the monkey bars. The blood rushes to your head and the pressure starts to increase. Only this was occurring when I was standing and during periods of exertion.

Initially, I was sent to a vascular specialist because the most prominent symptom was that my jugular veins would distend when this would happen. My upper torso, neck, arms, and face slowly started to swell and had a puffy appearance. I had an MRI which showed some sort of mass on and around my SVC. Cancer was the diagnosis that I think everyone thought I was expecting.

An interventional procedure was scheduled to try to balloon open my Superior Vena Cava (SVC) to see if they could establish blood flow. This was the defining moment for me in my diagnosis. The interventional radiologist who performed the procedure had studied in the Ohio River Valley area where fibrosing mediastinitis was very prevalent and had seen it before.

The procedure to open my SVC was unsuccessful, but he started my journey to the correct diagnosis. The surgical notes and report went through all the normal stuff, but it was the last sentence of that report that has changed my life: *possible fibrosing mediastinitis.*

Quickly, I was referred to an infectious disease doctor for treatment and understanding of histoplasmosis, the cause of this condition. I remember that visit like it was yesterday. I went alone and spent about four hours giving my life history. I remember thinking, *Man this guy knows more about me then my own mother.* I know many FM friends do not spend much time with infectious disease doctors, but we formed a bond that was unbreakable. He wanted to help me and I trusted him, a combination that served us well for seven years.

He introduced me to an infectious disease specialist at the University of Michigan. He trusted her and wanted to see how she could help me. The day I traveled the 120 miles to her office was a bit of a fog for me. My mother and brother were meeting us there and I had my two dearest friends with me for support. I'll never forget sitting in the meeting room, with a hopefulness that she was going to be able to help me and that she'd even heard of fibrosing mediastinitis.

In my mind, she was another angel who was looking over me that day and put me on the path to Vanderbilt. Literally, that night, I had packed my bags and we purchased three plane tickets. Our appointment with Dr. James Loyd was the next day at 1 pm.

So here we were now, sitting in the lobby of Vanderbilt Medical Center. Another step closer-- to what we were unsure-- but it was movement.

I was admitted and a series of tests were done to determine my status and condition. The results were a relief in the sense that we had a name for what was happening, but terrifying in regard to the unknown.

My SVC had narrowed and formed several blood clots. Amazingly, my body had developed collateral veins which were keeping me alive. My SVC was normally around 16 mm and was down to less than 1mm. My right pulmonary artery was approximately 50% blocked and half of my right lung was no longer functioning. Without intervention, my life, I am quite sure, would have been over.

I flew back to Michigan with the plan of taking blood thinners to try and break up the clots.* A surgery date was scheduled for December 17, 2004. It was around October 12, so I had about six weeks until I would head back down to Nashville for a stenting procedure by Dr. Thomas Doyle. Those six weeks, as I look back, are another story on coping and dealing with the fear of the unknown. Pema Chodron's book, The Places that Scare You: A Guide to Fearlessness in Difficult Times was on my bedside table along with my bible.

In those six weeks, I did manage to complete my last semester at Michigan State University to earn my MBA. I graduated on December 14, 2004 and turned around, just three days later, to head to Nashville.

Unfortunately, my clots had not broken up so the procedure also involved pulling out the clots through an access point in my jugular. Once the clots were removed, Dr. Doyle placed two stents in my SVC. The video is quite amazing to watch. The backflow before surgery and smooth blood flow after the stents were placed is incredible. I had measured my neck prior to the procedure and my neck diameter was reduced by two and a half inches after the procedure. The pressure in my head reduced drastically and when I woke the effects were felt immediately. *Relief.*

I returned to Michigan and went back to work. Life certainly didn't return to normal as hard as I tried to pick up where I left off. I was limited in my physical activity. I no longer pushed through those feelings of discomfort while exercising. I knew what it was now, so fear crippled me. Blood thinners became a part of my life, forever, a concept that weighed on me: *Forever.* But now it's just who I am.

A few months went by and I tried to normalize my life as much as possible I started to notice some trouble breathing. I contacted Vanderbilt and we decided to go in and stent my right pulmonary artery. The flow in the artery is much greater and stenting can be risky, but we felt like it was the right thing to do in order to keep blood flow to my right lung. Dr. Doyle was able to put two stents in the right PA in March 2005. That was my last interventional procedure to date.

During the last seven years, I've learned to live the best life I can. I have fibrosing mediastinitis and, as cliché as this may sound, it doesn't have me. It's certainly changed my life and given it certain direction, but I've lived. I've taken risks that were so important to me. I have an amazing husband and two miracle children that I was able to carry. I've learned to listen to my body and my heart and to trust in God. I accept the days that the disease wins and I submit. I still have periods of intense fear and grieving. I recognize that no one has a guarantee on tomorrow.

*Author's note: Blood thinners, such as Coumadin (warfarin) cannot break up existing clots. Coumadin is used to keep new clots from forming.

Terry

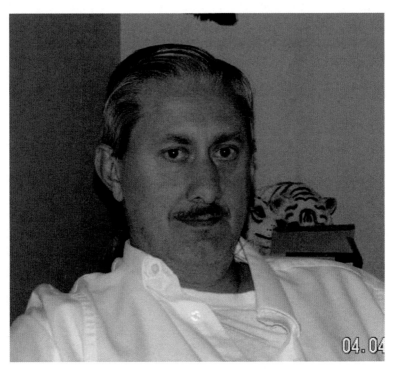

Terry was born in Grayson County, Kentucky. He's worked since he was fifteen years old and has rarely been sick except for seasonal allergies.

In December 2010, Terry began to notice his energy level was waning and he had some shortness of breath, which he contributed to smoking. His eyesight was changing and he felt that his arthritis was getting worse. By May, he was admitted to a Louisville hospital for three days with pneumonia.

His doctor did a CT scan and a bronchoscopy and diagnosed Terry, at the age of 49, with histo-related fibrosing mediastinitis. His symptoms were caused from occlusion of his left pulmonary artery and of his superior vena cava (SVC).

Terry went to Vanderbilt Hospital in Nashville where doctors attempted to insert a stent into his pulmonary artery. It was unsuccessful. They also tried to stent his SVC, but the opening was too narrow. Terry underwent thoracic surgery by Dr. Simon Maltais at the Vanderbilt University for replacement of his

SVC using a *PTFE Vascular Graft*. The graft failed within two weeks.

He reports that his health is a little better, but he still struggles with shortness of breath, fatigue, lightheadedness and body aches. He takes medications for his arthritis.

Terry can no longer work or do the things he used to do, like maintaining his home and yard. He becomes short of breath and fatigued. He doesn't sleep well. One of his frustrations lies in the fact that so few doctors know about his condition and he is never sure when he should go to the hospital for his symptoms.

Luke

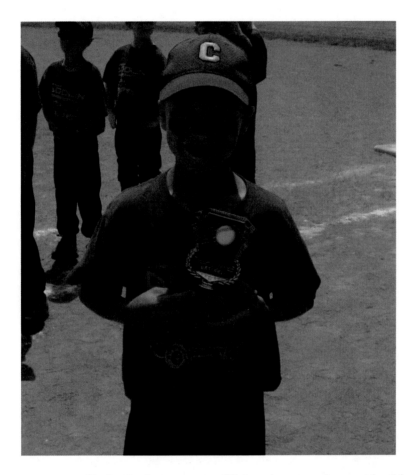

(Luke is the youngest FM patient to take part in this project. His story is told by his mother Kristy. Italics are referred to in the Glossary)

Luke is a twin born 11/3/2003 at 37 weeks, 6 lbs. 2 oz., 18.5 inches. No oxygen was necessary and he was born completely healthy.

He has grown up in central Illinois, about 25 miles east of Springfield. We live in a 100-year-old farm house surrounded by corn and soybean fields. We are not farmers and all the outbuildings were torn down before we saw the property so we are not sure what kind of animals were on the property in the past.

During infancy and toddler stage, Luke got sick with respiratory problems/ear infections probably three to four times during the winter months while his twin sister usually remained healthy. The family doctor said he got sick more often because he was a "white boy" and "white boys" usually are weaker health-wise.

His first diagnosis was mild asthma, then right middle lobe syndrome, persistent/recurrent pneumonia, granulomas disease, and now finally, post-histo FM.

During the winter of 2008 is when we first noticed something really was not normal. He was pretty much sick the entire fall/winter/spring. We thought maybe it was just because he had always stayed at home with me was never around a bunch of kids to be exposed to all the germs. He would run a fever of up to 103 or 104 that would last for a couple of days and then disappear. This would happen every week or two. The fever would come and go. If the fever lasted, I would take Luke to the doctor where he was either diagnosed with a viral infection, bronchitis or an ear infection and sent home on antibiotics. He was on so many antibiotics during this time that the doctor said he was running out of antibiotics to give him, especially since the first antibiotic usually did not work and he would then be placed on another.

The constant throughout this entire period of time was a wet cough that would bring up lots of mucus. This mucus was very thick and he would even blow bubbles with it. He would often cough until he vomited.

Luke was very active and never slowed down despite this. He played sports and would play through pain in his chest. He would wait until after games and climb in the car and then start crying about the pain, but he has never let any of his teammates see him hurting. We were amazed at his strength.

Spring 2009. After our constant inquires about the cough and why he was always getting sick, we were referred to a pediatric pulmonologist, Dr. Mark Johnson. Unfortunately, Dr. Johnson had too many patients and another doctor in his office could see Luke sooner.

We saw the other doctor. Although the fevers disappeared for the most part, Luke continued to have the cough with mucus and pleuritic pain with strenuous sporting activities. This lasted throughout the following visits, procedures, and tests. Occasionally the chest pain would occur even at rest.

June 17, 2009. Memorial Medical Center, Springfield, IL (MMC). Chest x-ray-Findings: Right middle lobe infiltrate (*an accumulation of something abnormal*) described on reports as a triangular focal opacity. Methacholine challenge-Findings: Airway sensitivity.

Middle of 2009- Diagnosed with mild asthma and started on inhalers: Flovent and Ventolin.

November 2009. Luke underwent a bronchoscopy and BAL (*bronchoalveolar lavage*) at St John's Outpatient Surgery Center (SJOSC), Springfield, Illinois in order to try and find the infiltrate that was on his chest x-rays.

Results: Lungs had mucus in his right middle lobe (RML) and lingula. *(a certain portion of the upper lobe of the left lung so named because it looks like a tongue)* They could not see an area of infiltrate. Culture results: *Streptococcus pneumoniae* and *Haemophilus influenzae*. (Both are bacteria, which unlike viruses or fungi, can be treated with antibiotics) Plan: Placed on Amoxicillin and increased Flovent dose.

2010-Saw doctor every three months for follow-up. We were told that he had right middle lobe syndrome for which the only treatment was inhalers.

Middle of 2010-Luke still continued to cough up a lot of mucus. We were told to change the way Luke was doing inhaler as he "must not be doing it right."

November 30, 2010- We saw Dr. Mark Johnson. He was very concerned that nothing had been followed up on since his last bronchoscopy. Dr. Johnson started things going to figure out what was going on.

1. Ordered chest x-ray

2. Ordered blood work to check for antibodies and immune system

3. Ordered sweat chloride test. (A test used to diagnose cystic fibrosis, a condition unrelated to FM)

November 30, 2010-(MMC) Got chest x-ray which showed the opacity and blood work which was essentially normal.

December 2, 2010- Luke had a sweat chloride test at MMC. The results were within normal limits.

December 7, 2010- Luke underwent a bronchoscopy at St. John's. His lungs were full of pus/mucus. The physician had to remove the scope and camera twelve times to clean it so he could continue. Luke came home and ran a fever of 104.5. Culture results: *Streptococcus pneumoniae* and *Haemophilus influenzae*. He was placed on antibiotics once again.

December 23, 2010- Another follow-up with Dr. Johnson. He still had coughing so he was placed on another antibiotic. The diagnosis at this time was recurrent/persistent pneumonia.

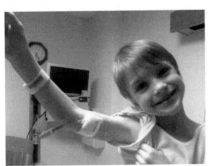

Luke shows off his PICC line

January 12, 2011 Chest x-ray at MMC and follow-up with Dr. Johnson. Infiltrate still there. Luke was admitted to MMC for 23-hour observation for insertion of PICC line (*an intravenous line inserted into a large vein*) and to begin IV antibiotics. He was sent home on an every eight hour schedule.

While in the hospital, we had a consultation with an ENT (ears/nose/throat) physician. Dr. Johnson wanted them to perform a rigid scope bronchoscopy and ciliary (*tiny hair-like projections in the lungs that help keep the lung free of debris*) biopsy. After eight days, he had to be taken off the IV antibiotics due to a whole body rash and was placed back on oral antibiotics.

February 21, 2011- Luke underwent another bronchoscopy at St. John's with BAL and ciliary biopsy performed by ENT, Dr. Sandra Ettema, in Springfield, Illinois. He was again admitted for 23-hour observation. Every part of his lungs was full of mucus and pus. Dr. Ettema had never seen anything like it. She said that by the looks of his lungs he should be disabled and unable to do anything. She described the secretions as very thick with some parts almost like concrete. Specimens were sent off to lab for culture. A ciliary biopsy was sent to Mayo Clinic. A barium swallow was performed and was normal. (*A test to assess the esophagus*) He was then set up with physical therapy to help with his breathing. He was sent home on mucomyst nebulizers. (*A medication used to break up mucus*)

February 24, 2011- Luke began physical therapy. His breathing muscles were weak. He would often hold his breath during regular breathing and when performing strenuous activity. The therapist taught us breathing techniques and chest percussion to use to help clear out the mucus.

We met with an infectious disease doctor who told us the cultures from his bronchoscopy were not significant and the ciliary biopsy was normal.

We requested that Luke see another doctor. We were referred to St. Louis Children's Hospital at Washington University. By this time, Luke's cough and mucus production had improved significantly, but they were still present.

March 21, 2011- Luke saw a doctor in St. Louis. Luke's pulmonary function testing (PFT) looked very good. The doctor repeated the sweat chloride test and again and it came back normal. We followed up a month later.

March 25, 2011- Luke had a CT scan of chest with contrast at MMC. The findings included atelectasis of his right middle lobe, infrahilar (*the area where the windpipe divides into the two lungs*) calcified adenopathy (*enlarged lymph node*), 3.5 mm nodule in the right middle lobe. We were given the diagnosis of granulomas disease of the chest. (*an area of tissue damaged by infection or injury*)

By this point, the coughing was only occurring rarely. The mucus production had stopped. We followed up in St. Louis and they agreed with the granulomas diagnosis and recommended he follow up in a year with another chest CT.

Luke has remained fairly healthy. He is very active in sports and still gets pleuritic pains if we do not give him albuterol before practice/games. Occasionally he still gets pains during rest.

July 2012. Luke was able to get switched to Dr. Mark Johnson with SIU in Springfield, Illinois for his one year follow-up. Dr. Johnson reviewed everything from the past years. He looked at the CT scan from a year prior and immediately saw what he felt was fibrosing mediastinitis, most likely from histoplasmosis, but ordered blood work to confirm. He also ordered another CT scan. After reviewing the blood work and both CT scans, he confirmed the diagnosis of post-histo FM. The CT report now included multiple calcified mediastinal subcarinal and right hilar lymph nodes, the opacity now with chunky calcifications measuring about 3.5 cm and the 3 mm lung nodule in the right middle lobe. Spirometry testing has been fairly normal. A V/Q scan (ventilation/perfusion scan) was performed which was normal.

Dr. Johnson performed another bronchoscopy and this time Luke's lungs were clear of mucus. It was discovered that the opening to his right middle lobe was reduced by sixty percent.

The plan for Luke is to monitor him with bronchoscopes yearly, as needed, and CT scans every two years as long as he is asymptomatic. He still has his inhalers and mostly just uses his albuterol as needed. He is on no other meds or oxygen.

His health today is the same as when diagnosed, but much better than at the beginning of our four year journey.

The biggest frustration is no one has heard of FM and we have to educate everyone we meet. Luke is Dr. Johnson's second patient and youngest patient he has seen. Fortunately, he follows Dr. James Loyd's work.

It took four years and many diagnoses to get to where Luke is now with a diagnosis of post-histo FM at the age of eight. Dr. James Loyd at Vanderbilt in Nashville gave us a little bit of hope at the FM Conference in August 2012. After talking to us, he seemed very skeptical that Luke, because of his young age, actually had fibrosing mediastinitis. He thought, perhaps, Luke had some complication from histoplasmosis, but not FM. However, after reviewing his CT scans and other tests and reports he confirmed that Luke does indeed have post-histo FM.

We have no idea as to Luke's prognosis. No one has been able to answer because no one knows. I am grateful though to hear a doctor say "I don't know" rather than to hear them guessing. It's better to have no idea than a wrong prognosis which is dismal. The only thing Dr. Loyd and Dr. Johnson have said is that Luke's major structure affected is the right middle lobe, the smallest portion of the lung, which is good.

We are still concerned about whether more needs to be looked into with his blood flow. Our pulmonologist says since Luke is doing okay and keeping up with his friends, further study probably isn't necessary. However, we are not comfortable with this answer and we plan to get him evaluated by a cardiologist.

Luke is an amazing child. He is strong willed and a pain in the butt at times, but extremely loving and hard driven. He doesn't know failure nor does he allow it to happen. He has been amazing throughout this. I cannot believe a child can be as strong as he is. Health care professionals tell us often how he handles things much better than many adults. He never questions or complains, no matter what test he was undergoing. If a doctor or nurse told him to do something, he did it.

It broke our hearts as he was being wheeled down to get a PICC line and looked at us with tears in his eyes asking, "Why does everything happen to me?" and when he whispered in my ear as the doctor was giving us the FM diagnosis, "Am I going to die?" We have taught him the name of his diagnosis in case of an emergency and we aren't around. We are, however, trying to protect him from finding out the possibilities of the outcome of this disease. We want him to remain "normal" in his own eyes. Although, after the conference, we told him the doctor said the fibrous tissue was like wood so now he likes to say he has a wooden lung. He also found it quite amusing that when the doctor taps on his lungs, it makes a thud over the right side. He tries to do it at home to show off, but he hasn't been able to figure out how.

Luke is a typical boy. We have to be very vigilant in trying to keep him healthy. It is difficult to do when at this age kids are--as I describe them--little germ magnets. Hand washing is stressed continuously and we are constantly on him about putting things into his mouth. He drives us insane because he touches everything where ever we go. He always has to "just see what that is." Hand sanitizer is the first thing he gets when he climbs back into the car. With FM, every cold he catches has the potential to turn into pneumonia and end up as a hospitalization. Flu shots for the whole family are no longer an option, but a must.

Felicia

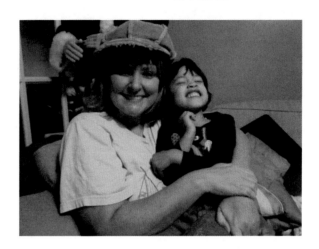

Felicia, who is now fifty, began having shortness of breath, fatigue, and frequent lung infections when she was twenty five. She grew up in New Lexington, Ohio.

Her initial diagnoses included a congenital hypoplastic pulmonary artery (*an underdeveloped artery from birth*) and a pulmonary embolism. She was told her shortness of breath was due to being overweight.

She was finally diagnosed, at the Ohio State University, with right pulmonary artery occlusion from post-histo fibrosing mediastinitis at the age of forty seven. Felicia was never given a prognosis for her FM.

"My biggest fear is the unknown."

She had a job, but fatigue and shortness of breath keep her from full-time employment.

"My son carries the groceries and my husband does laundry because I can't carry things upstairs."

"I want to run, play tennis, swim, and paint my house," Felicia says, but she is reluctant to pursue treatment. "I want to have stents, but I am afraid they might not work like they do for others. I see the problems that can occur. I feel torn whether to stay the way I am or take a chance and maybe get better."

Felicia says her biggest frustration with her condition is "having a disease that others cannot see." She also struggles financially because of medical bills and the inability to work full-time.

Recently, Felicia was told by doctors at Vanderbilt that stenting her pulmonary artery was impossible. She is currently seeking second opinions.

Mary Ellen

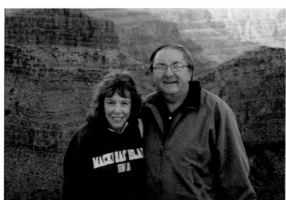

Thank you to my family and friends for their love, support, and encouragement through my journey with FM

Mary Ellen was born and raised in Watertown, Wisconsin.

She went to college in Whitewater, WI and spent some vacations near her mother, who had moved to Winona, Minnesota, along the Mississippi River where Mary Ellen worked at a YMCA camp. Mary Ellen moved to Sturgeon Bay, Wisconsin in 1978 and has lived there for 34 years.

Before Mary Ellen was diagnosed with FM, she had fever, night sweats, and continuous coughing.

"I felt like I had fluid in my lungs or heart because I couldn't lie down in bed and slept many nights in a recliner." She also had facial swelling and *atrial fibrillation*.

Mary Ellen was treated at North Shore Medical Center (now named Ministry Door County Medical Center) with help by Bellin Hospital in Green Bay "My family doctor sent me to a different doctor at the clinic, an internist with expertise in pulmonary problems. He thought it was possibly *sarcoidosis*. Chest x-rays did not show anything, but pulmonary function tests, CT scan, bronchoscopy with a lung biopsy, and mediastinoscopy with paratracheal lymph node biopsy led to her diagnosis of histo-related FM in May 2008.

"When we found out it was FM the doctor informed me that it was very rare and that I would most likely be the only case that he'd see in his lifetime. I was fortunate that he was willing to learn more about it and talk to other doctors at various clinics."

Mary Ellen's tests were evaluated by Marshfield Clinic in Marshfield, Wisconsin and Mayo Clinic in Rochester, Minnesota. Dr. Loyd from Vanderbilt Medical Center reviewed her CT scan.

"My FM affects my airways. There is proliferation of abnormal tissue in the mediastinum that surrounds my airways on both sides. It affects the mediastinum, hila, and tracheobronchial tree. There is severe narrowing with possible occlusion of the right middle lobe bronchus. The doctors are not able to put stents in this area to open it up. The lungs are showing a ground glass opacity and consolidation in both lungs."

"At first I was told that 'it would burn itself out' and that I would have to deal with the problems it left, but that I shouldn't get any worse. They said that it wasn't a progressive disease, but that hasn't been the case. Now I deal with each problem as they come up. My prognosis isn't very good, but I am trying to keep a positive attitude."

"FM has been taking over my life. It is very difficult for me to plan any activities because I do not know how I will feel from day to day."

Mary Ellen was a special education teacher for thirty three years. She worked with students with cognitive, developmental, and behavioral challenges.

"I never really sat down at work. I was involved with the students and would not ask my assistants to do any tasks that I wouldn't do myself. We worked on academics, vocational tasks, went on community trips, and worked on social skills in functional settings."

She tried to work for a period of time after her symptoms began.

"At first I just coughed a lot."

When she coughed so much that she began vomiting, Mary Ellen found it difficult to work.

"The students were distracted by my coughing. Then I started having a hard time walking through the school and I couldn't carry anything or even pull a cart without getting short of breath. I couldn't run to keep up with the students. It was difficult to lift items to the shelves or to do the trips and activities of daily living. I was very tired just trying to get through the day. It was getting harder to focus and complete the paperwork that needed to be done."

"The fall after I retired I began to have trouble talking and found out I had a paralyzed vocal cord which, on top of everything else, would have made it impossible to do my job."

Mary Ellen experiences severe shortness of breath with exertion, lower extremity swelling, chest and upper back pain, weakness and a cough.

"I can no longer work or even volunteer at this time."

Mary Ellen loved being a special education teacher. "It was who I was. I was very emotional for months after school started. I went to the Humane Society to get a cat because I was so sad and lonely. She has been a great lap cat, therapist and companion."

"I can't do daily household tasks such as cleaning or laundry for any amount of time. It is very frustrating. Grocery shopping is very difficult, but if I try to buy some things it is hard, if not impossible, to carry packages up our stairs."

"The saddest and most difficult thing for me is not being able to care for our grandchildren because I can't keep up with them or walk up the stairs very easily to help them get their baths and go to bed.

"Recently, I have had a paralyzed left vocal cord which they believe is due to the FM causing laryngeal nerve paralysis. Reading stories to our three year-old granddaughter is even too challenging. I love to talk to people so it has been very difficult for me"

"I can't exercise. I used to go to the YMCA for classes. I had lost quite a bit of weight, but I am gaining it back partly because of the prednisone I have to take. Last summer, I fell three times and cracked by pelvis. My bones are getting weaker most likely due to the prednisone that I have been on for a couple of years." *

"I now have home oxygen which I sleep with every night and I need to take it with me when I travel. I also have a bi-pap sleep machine, a nebulizer, and take a variety of medication. I do not travel light!"

"I feel bad for my husband because he has to do so much and works so hard. I am very grateful he is here. I don't know what I would do without him!"

"This is a very lonely disease and even though you do not feel well you have to do a lot of research on your own and treatment is trial and error. I am so grateful for meeting people on the internet and through Facebook that have this disease. They have been so helpful and understanding."

*Long term use of Prednisone may cause bone density loss.

Carol

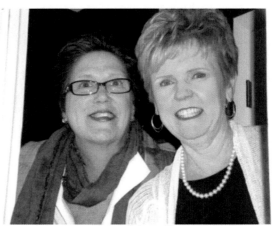

Carol (lt), and her partner Diane

Carol's lung problems started several years ago. In 1971, she had hemoptysis, underwent an angiogram and was diagnosed with a blood clot in her right pulmonary artery. She had Heparin injections and was started on a regimen of Coumadin for a year, requiring blood tests every 3-4 weeks.

"After a year, I was sent on my way," she says. "During my early thirties things were quiet. I was doing ten miles a day on a stationary Schwinn Airdine bike and religiously worked out with free weights three times a week. Then I started to have severe palpitation. They were so severe that I truly thought I would die." In retrospect, Carol noticed facial swelling during that time.

She went to the cardiologist several times. "My heart checked out just beautifully," she says. The cardiologist put her on Lopressor for her palpitations.

"One cardiologist noticed a varicose vein running across my stomach. He called his nurse over to look at it. 'I've never seen anything like this before,' he said. He hooked me up to an EKG and my heart was going wild. In hindsight, you would think he would have sent me to a vascular specialist. I truly think women are not treated equally to men when it comes to heart issues," Carol says.

"I had a very fulfilling and successful career. I worked full time and got my undergraduate degree at night. My business was in publishing. I worked from Maine to Florida and out to the Ohio border. I was constantly flying, driving rental cars and sleeping in hotels."

Over the years she developed lung pain, shortness of breath, palpitations, and blackouts. She noticed her stamina declining and had bouts of pneumonia.

"My health started to deteriorate in my late 40's and early 50's. Something was going terribly wrong. I was losing my edge and becoming very tired. I would arrive at a Trade Show and would walk into Jacob Javits Convention Center in New York or McCormick Place in Chicago and I would almost cry. It was so overwhelming. My memory was affected. I would forget flights or would arrive a day early to an appointment."

Carol stopped exercising and could not function with her day-to-day expectations. She would say to Diane, her partner, "I just can't get though the demands of what my job requires of me... or anything else for that matter." She would take off her bra at 2pm and sneak out of the shows to rest. "The bra was occluding part of my circulatory system. I cannot wear one to this day. The pain from those collateral veins, similar to varicose veins, is excruciating, not to mention that it blocks off the circulation going to my heart since my superior vena cava is totally occluded."

"One day, while traveling, I was putting my luggage in the overhead compartment of the plane and tore my left rotator cuff. Or so we thought. The MRI showed a full thickness tear. I went in to get it fixed and on the operating table I woke up, gasping for air. They said, 'Don't worry, Carol. Everything will be OK' and I went back under."

"In the recovery room, an anesthesiologist rushed to my bed side and told me, 'You have to carry a card that says you must have a fiberoptic laryngeal tube to go down your throat when you have surgery.' She gave me no reason. I was out of it from the surgery."

Carol later found out that she had no tear in her shoulder, but surgeons aspirated some blood from the area. She was sent home and nothing more was said.

"After all of that, I developed a swelling of my left lymph node. I went to my primary doctor and he sent me for a CT scan. My life was derailed from there."

At age 55, Carol was diagnosed with post- histo fibrosing mediastinitis.

"I had test after test and second opinions, all the while having horrible pain in my right lung. My upper right rib felt as if it was snapped in half. All of my veins are going every which way. One runs left and should be running right. This is my circulation." Carol describes her collateral circulation, a typical development with people with FM, especially those with superior vena cava occlusion.

Carol's FM affects her SVC, her right pulmonary artery, esophagus, airway, and heart. She has left lung calcifications, as well, that are being watched by her physicians.

"My doctor always has time for me. We sit and talk and he answers all my questions. When we first met, he sat down with me and said my CT showed that my superior vena cava was totally obstructed. He said it was as if you had a garden hose and someone poured cement down the hose then packed a big baseball of cement around it. I also have occlusion of my innominate (*brachiocephalic*) vein, left lung, and right pulmonary artery."

Carol was sent from Thomas Jefferson University Hospital in Philadelphia to Mayo Clinic for specialized care. "When I explained my symptoms, they doubted that I had fibrosing mediastinitis, coming from the east coast. After several more tests, they came to the conclusion that I did, indeed, have FM."

"The doctors at the Mayo Clinic debated whether or not to remove my right lung and do a spiral vein graft for my superior vena cava. They agreed that doing it would be too dangerous and I could possibly be dead within the year."

The plan is to watch and wait. Carol lives with pain every day. She has gotten a lot of help from Thomas Jefferson University Pain Center in Philadelphia. "Thank God for them. They took the time to understand the disease. I really don't know what I would do if I had to live with the levels of pain I experience. Even with all of my meds, I am still in pain every day. I can tolerate the pain a bit more."

Doctors are looking at Carol's clotting issues and wondering if she has a hyper-coagulation disorder. They are not clear whether or not she is chronically thrombosing. (*clotting*)

She had a cardiac catheterization that revealed several myocardial infarctions (*heart attacks*) that have left her with necrotic (*dead*) heart muscle. "I have blood flow through my heart as if the mighty Mississippi has gone down to a trickling stream."

She has coronary artery spasms for which she takes nitroglycerine and must lie down to get her feet above heart level. If that doesn't help her, she goes to the hospital immediately.

She routinely goes through EKG's, echocardiograms, lung tests, ultrasounds of her extremities, and an annual CT scan. She has difficulty with food passing through her esophagus and has recently discovered that her esophagus is inadequate, causing her to choke. She is scheduled for a procedure to stretch the esophagus. "This is just another symptom in my FM journey."

"I have a wonderful partner and wife, Diane, and lovely people around me. They do anything I need them to do. I try to do some light cleaning or loading the dishwasher, things like that, but I feel myself changing every day. Lifting my grandchildren is harder. If they lean against my side, the vascular pain from my collaterals is terrible. As I said, my career is over. I loved it so much. I'm not trying to blow my horn, but I was good at it."

"I just lost my rock, my mother, Catherine Valaitis. She would follow-up with our FM group to encourage them daily. She was 87 when she passed on February 12, 2012."

Angela

Angela grew up and lives in Lauderdale County, Tennessee, an endemic area for histoplasmosis.

The first symptom that Angela noticed before her FM diagnosis was that she had prominent veins across her chest. "My chest looked like a road map." She also had facial swelling and shortness of breath, all the hallmarks of SVC syndrome. She saw a vein doctor who ordered a CT scan. He then sent her to a pulmonologist, Dr. Michael Smith, in Memphis, Tennessee.

In 2008, at the age of twenty seven, Angela was diagnosed with histo fibrosing mediastinitis and had a stent placed in her superior vena cava at Baptist Memorial Hospital in Memphis.

Angela says she feels a little better since her stent placement, but she fears the unknown that comes with having FM.

Brenda H.

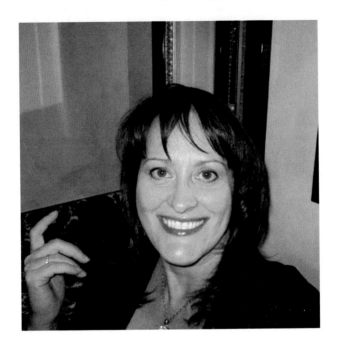

Brenda grew up on a farm with chickens and cows in Ontario, Canada. She sold vegetables at a farmers' market as a teenager. She also worked at a race track.

"I had mononucleosis at sixteen and was very sick for a year. Then I was anemic and had to take iron shots. Shortly after that, I developed a virus in my heart, according to a cardiologist. My heart was literally thumping in my chest."

In 1990 and 1991, she visited Slovenia where she toured huge caves. She recalls the floors being covered with orange bat guano, a known source of the histoplasmosis spore.

Before Brenda was diagnosed with fibrosing mediastinitis she was working as a financial planner. During that time, she felt short of breath, had frequent anxiety and panic attacks, and felt her heart was racing. She had frequent bouts of bronchitis and lung infections. Blood tests showed that she had antibodies for scleroderma and lupus. She was treated with antibiotics, but never seemed to get better.

In 1996 Brenda went for in-vitro fertilization to try to conceive.

"I specifically remember when I did the in-vitro fertilization that the nurse questioned me, 'do you have any problems with your lungs?' I told her that I had recurring lung infections because I didn't know about the condition yet. I always wondered if in-vitro fertilization treatment worsened my condition."

After the second unsuccessful attempt, she developed a cough which would produce severe coughing fits. "One morning I coughed up a big chunk of blood," she said.

That's when the medical investigations began.

In 1997, Brenda's FM was discovered on a CT scan at the St. Joseph's Hospital in Hamilton, Ontario. She was 35 years old. She has possible occlusion of her superior vena cava and of her left pulmonary artery. She has been told her condition cannot be improved with interventions, although she is seeing a cardiologist in the upcoming months who, she hopes, will shed some light on her condition.

Brenda says she has no energy and her bad days far outweigh the good. "On good days I overdo it and the next day I have no energy." She has frequent shortness of breath, chest pain, body aches, fatigue, and a racing heart. "My heart will beat 140 times a minute at rest," she says. She still uses steroid inhalers for asthma.

FM has affected Brenda's life drastically. She has difficulty planning because she never knows how she is going to feel. "I am leery of socializing during flu season, mostly because a lot of the antibiotics don't work for me," she says. "I don't deal with stress well." Similar to other FM patients' reports, Brenda has more difficulty with hot and humid weather. "People look at me and say, 'Gee, you look so great…there's nothing wrong with you.' That's the hardest thing. No one knows what's going on inside."

Brenda's recent tests for lupus and scleroderma have turned up negative. "I don't know what my FM progression is," she says. "I don't want to have any more dyes in my body so I haven't had any CAT scans in a while."

Brenda reports other conditions: fibromyalgia, degenerative disc disease, end plate sclerosis of the spine, chronic fatigue syndrome. Some of these conditions have been classified as autoimmune. She also tells me her mother was a heavy smoker when her mother was pregnant with her. Whether there is a connection to FM and other autoimmune diseases is not yet clear.

Lori

Lori grew up in Milledgeville, Georgia. As a child, she was told she had asthma. In late 2011, Lori began to experience fatigue, severe shortness of breath, flu-like symptoms, fever, and chest pain and was diagnosed with pneumonia.

In January 2012, Lori, 31, underwent a bronchoscopy and a Chamberlain procedure, a type of mediastinoscopy, at the Georgia Health Sciences Medical Center in Augusta, Georgia. She had three large masses removed. Her airway and left pulmonary artery are affected by histo-related fibrosing mediastinitis.

In spite of interventions, Lori still experiences shortness of breath, severe pain, fatigue, and high blood pressure. She is told by her doctors that her condition is likely to worsen. She attributes her anxiety and related panic attacks to her FM diagnosis.

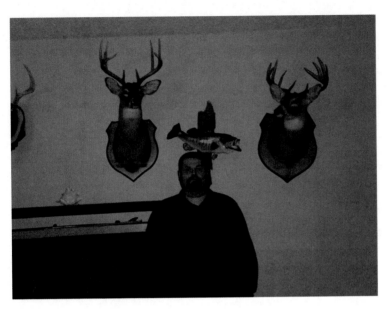

Shane

Shane is a 40 year-old man living in Indianapolis, Indiana. He spent his summers in Illinois and Kentucky. He could have contracted his histoplasmosis in any of those places, but, like many others, Shane's histo went undiagnosed. Shane had episodes of hemoptysis nine years before his diagnosis of fibrosing mediastinitis.

In 2010, Shane began having chest pains, increased shortness of breath and a cough. He was also fatigued and had severe headaches, especially with exertion. After a gamut of routine cardiac tests, doctors told Shane he had asthma related to cigarette smoking.

He stopped smoking, but Shane's symptoms did not subside and further tests at the IU Health Center in Indianapolis, including a CT angiogram *(dye is injected into the body during a CT scan to watch blood flow)*, showed that Shane's right pulmonary artery was completely occluded. He has had difficulty obtaining the care he needs for many reasons. Shane's pulmonologist told his employer that he might have difficulty with hot and humid weather. His employer decided Shane would not be able to perform his job adequately. While he was on leave (FMLA) for his illness, his employer terminated him. As a result, he lost his medical insurance and has become bankrupt due to medical bills. He struggles emotionally because of the toll his diagnosis has taken.

Shane's quality of life has diminished. Once an avid hunter and fisherman, he is limited by his ongoing chest pain and shortness of breath and requires supplemental oxygen. His occluded artery leaves him feeling fatigued and he says he "feels useless."

Because Shane has no insurance and is currently in flux about medical assistance, he can do nothing but wait...and hope. There are very few physicians who would be willing or able to help Shane with his arterial occlusion. The doctors he has seen have told him that his condition is irreversible. He is not financially equipped to seek the medical help he knows may be available to help him to improve his quality of life. He is hoping Medicare will kick in by the beginning of 2013.

From what I can gather, Shane's illness has left him feeling emasculated, both mentally and physically.

"A healthy sex life is a must and I find it difficult because I get so short of breath."

He's lost his way of living and providing for his family and the stress of watching his bills pile up is draining. He's embarrassed by his oxygen tank and feels that people may perceive him as lazy or weak.

"I can't even mow my own lawn or keep up house maintenance without paying someone or talking a friend into helping."

Bill

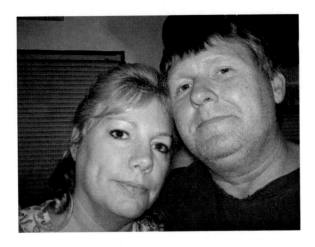

Bill was born in Hartford City, Indiana where he was raised, living most of his life on a farm.

Bill began having chest pain, lightheadedness, dizziness, and difficulty breathing. He had episodes of hemoptysis (*coughing up blood*) and syncope (*passing out*). Chronically fatigued, he sought medical attention and was found to have *pericardial effusions*.

The heart is surrounded by a membrane, called a pericardium or pericardial sac, for protection. In some conditions, fluid or blood can build up between lining of the sac and the heart muscle. This puts pressure on the heart muscle that may cause the heart to fail as a pump. Bill had developed four effusions and had them drained. Finally, his physician told him he should have the pericardium removed, a surgical procedure called a *pericardiectomy*.

In 2009 Bill, at the age of 43, underwent the surgery at the Lutheran Hospital in Ft. Wayne, Indiana. Thoracic surgeon, William Deschner, found the underlying cause of Bill's pericardial effusions: fibrosing mediastinitis related to an earlier histoplasmosis infection. Bill grew up right in the heart of the histoplasmosis endemic area.

Unfortunately, Bill's FM is widespread. In spite of an eight hour surgery to try to eliminate some of the fibrosis, Bill still has involvement of his heart, lungs, and esophagus.

He has been treated with a drug regimen of steroids and itraconazole, an anti-fungal agent that, although has not been shown to help with people with FM, may be effective for those with an acute histoplasmosis infection. His physician has told him that his FM is progressing and has given him a grim prognosis: six months to two years.

Bill says that he's not afraid of dying, but is deeply concerned about his wife, children, and grandchildren. He wonders how they must feel knowing that they will lose him in the near future.

"My wife, kids and grandbabies are what hurts me the most. My wife works nights and wonders whether or not I'll be here or if she'll find me dead in the morning. FM did not just change my life, but all our lives."

Bill treasures his wife Gladys' devotion. "She's there for all of us," he says. "Sometimes she gets run down taking care of me. I owe it all to her and wouldn't have made it this long without her."

Bill has been unable to work. He says that he has bad days when he can't get out of bed due to extreme fatigue and he is unable to travel far from home. He has severe chest pains, "like a vice" and has trouble breathing. He has headaches and some difficulty with thought processes and forgetfulness.

"Sometimes I'm in bed for days. I just want to be able to enjoy nice days."

Melissa M.

Melissa is a forty year-old woman who was born in Fall Branch, Tennessee. She began to have severe headaches, fatigue and her eyes and neck began to swell. She also had *vertigo* when she would bend over and stand back up.

Her doctor told her she had asthma and then told her she had coccidiomycosis (Valley Fever), a fungal disease that is endemic in the western United States.

At the age of 35, she changed doctors and discovered the cause of her symptoms: occlusion of her superior vena cava as a result of fibrosing mediastinitis secondary to a histoplasmosis infection (*at least physicians were right in that she had a fungal infection*).

At Vanderbilt Children's Hospital in Nashville, TN, Melissa has had placement of six stents in her SVC over a three year period. She takes Coumadin to keep her blood thin.

She lives in Kingsport, Tennessee with her husband and still works 12-hour shifts, but they wear her out and she still has shortness of breath. Her husband, she says, is her "rock" and the illness has brought them closer together.

Although Melissa still has headaches and some swelling, she says that her FM is stable. "I just have to watch my symptoms."

Brenda W.

Brenda grew up and lives in Missouri with her husband.

In early 2006, when she was 43, Brenda began to have pain in her right chest, shortness of breath, and a chronic cough. She had trouble sleeping and was gaining weight.

Doctors initially told her she had a condition called hereditary hemorrhagic telangiectasia (HHT aka Osler-Weber-Rendu syndrome), a genetic condition where a person can develop abnormal blood vessels called arteriovenous malformations (AVMs) in several areas of the body. If they are on the skin, they are called telangiectasias. The abnormal blood vessels can also develop in the brain, lungs, liver, intestines, or other areas. Symptoms of HHT include shortness of breath, but also include frequent nosebleeds in children, gastrointestinal bleeding, seizures or small strokes (*due to bleeding in the brain*).

In August 2006, Brenda underwent a pulmonary angiogram and an echocardiogram and was diagnosed with histo-FM at Barnes Jewish Hospital in St. Louis, Missouri. She has occlusion of her superior pulmonary vein that involves the left upper lobe and the pulmonary vein of her right upper lobe with segmental branches of the right lower lobe. She also has occlusion of her right pulmonary artery.

At Vanderbilt Hospital in Nashville, doctors were able to stent her superior pulmonary vein. She takes blood thinners daily and is on oxygen all the time. She also takes pain medications for chest pain.

"I have shortness of breath all the time. When I try to clean my house I am worn out for days afterwards. I'm not sure my husband understands this disease at all and he feels that I should do everything I used to do. It's just not possible and it sometimes puts a strain on our marriage. I have a really hard time losing weight because I can't exercise like I want. Plus, I seem to catch everything I come in contact with."

Like most people with fibrosing mediastinitis, Brenda expresses finances and the lack of information as sources of her frustration. She is on disability because of her FM. "The Medicare is about useless," she says. "If it was better I would not have to put out money for other insurance. My husband works, but, like a lot of other people, we live paycheck to paycheck. We can't afford a new car and I have trouble getting to doctors' appointments."

Because Brenda's fibrosing mediastinitis is bilateral, meaning that she has involvement of both her right and left lung, her physician has also given her a poor prognosis. "They said that if it starts growing again that it would not take long for it to choke everything off. My right lung only has a quarter of its function. I keep praying that things will get better."

Rick

"I have lived most of my life in histoplasmosis endemic areas and was, like most people, oblivious to it." Rick grew up in Northwestern Illinois, an endemic area for histoplasmosis. "Looking back, I can think of numerous events and locations where I could have become infected with histoplasmosis. Would I have worn a respirator had I known? I don't know. But people reading this are now faced with that dilemma. There is almost nothing good that comes from breathing in dusty environments or any place that has been contaminated with bat or bird poop."

Rick's battle with fibrosing mediastinitis began in his early twenties.

"During the summer of 1984, I lost a lot of weight and had night sweats. During the fall, I started coughing up blood periodically. On Christmas Eve, I went to see a local doctor who did a chest x-ray that identified a mediastinal mass of unknown entity."

"On January 12, 1985, I was admitted to University of Iowa Hospitals in Iowa City Iowa. I had a CT scan with contrast and then a bronchoscopy to obtain a biopsy. I recall being told the mass was too vascular and could not be cut out for fear of uncontrolled bleeding. A right *thoracotomy* was scheduled for the next day to obtain and identify the mass. This was completed and the results showed scar tissue with evidence of histoplasmosis."

The fibrosing mediastinitis that Rick has involves his superior vena cava (SVC), right pulmonary artery, esophagus, airway, and heart.

"Initially, in 1985, I had one grapefruit size mass with bronchial involvement. By 1995, a second mass, further up the neck, appeared that was affecting the right internal jugular and other nearby structures. The original mass was now nearly doubled in size and was occluding the SVC, the right pulmonary artery, and the azygos vein. (A blood vessel that's located along the right side of the thoracic vertebral column). The mass also surrounded the esophagus as well as compressed my trachea."

Today, Rick lives in Virginia with his wife. He is on oxygen all the time. He takes a host of medications, including anti-hypertensives, diuretics, anti-depressants, and pain medicine. He has undergone cardiac ablation, cardioversion, and heart reconstructive surgery on his right atrium. Surgeons created a new tube/conduit to his left brachiocephalic vein and then used a Gortex patch to rebuild Rick's right atrium. He has also had two stent placements, along with numerous other tests.

Rick has been one of the people instrumental in getting patients involved with their disease and care. He has been an online presence for a number of years. He says he gets frustrated with the lack of correct understanding many patients have about their disease.

"Many people don't understand the difference between histoplasmosis and fibrosing mediastinitis."

He also expresses concern about the isolation many patients have in dealing with FM and its difficulties. Rick has lived with FM longer than anyone else I interviewed for this book.

"In 1985, they told me I had only months to live. In 1995, they told me the same thing. Then, in 2002, the doctors asked me, 'You know what happens when you have FM?' I said, 'What? You die?' The doctor answered, 'Yes.'"

"Doctors at Duke University Hospitals say I am going to live a good long time. They don't elaborate about quality of life, but that is what we keep focusing on. Of course, there are always treatments for the symptoms that come along."

FM has made life challenging for Rick and his family.

"The appointments, the bills, the worries about procedures and the unknown after unknown have made it challenging, but life is a challenge anyway. This one is most definitely different from what I had in mind, but I don't know that it is any worse. I have had to work hard and believe all people should. My wife has been my champion all along and I'm glad to have her on my side."

Sheila

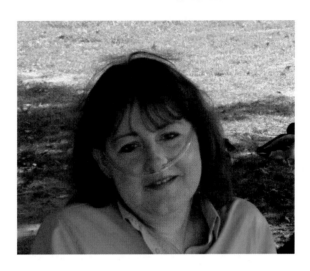

This is from a blog that Sheila kept and is in her own words, written December 5, 2007.

I really wanted to share with everyone the whole story of my lung disease from the very beginning.

It started about twelve years ago, when I was in my early twenties. It seemed like all of a sudden I started getting sick a lot. In a matter of just a few months I was hospitalized three separate times: twice for pneumonia and once for pleurisy. I also had my tonsils and adenoids removed. Well, needless to say I got tired of being sick so I sat down with the doctor and asked them to do some kind of testing to see why I was getting sick all the time. I was tired of them just fixing me because I would always just get sick again.

They sent me for tests and told me that there was something showing up on my lungs and they needed to do a needle biopsy to find out what they were dealing with. They told me, at the time, they believed it to be cancer. So, I went for the needle biopsy and they couldn't get what they needed to make a diagnosis.

Then they decided to do an open lung biopsy. I had the operation. I was in the hospital for two weeks. I still am not sure how I survived that surgery. Anyway, when they got the results back from the biopsy it turns out that I had a rare lung disease called fibrosing mediastinitis caused by a super human response to histoplasmosis. They treated the histoplasmosis and told me there wasn't anything they could do for the FM (Fibrosing Mediastinitis) because there wasn't a cure. They said that the Mayo Clinic was doing research and if they ever came up with anything someone would call me.

Please try to remember that I was a young girl in my early twenties and had very little experience with doctors or anything medical. They did not act as though this was a terrible disease that would continue to grow. I was never followed up with in regards to this disease again. I went back to life as usual.

I noticed, over the years, that my breathing was getting worse, but I thought that was just from losing part of the right lung (taken during the open lung biopsy years earlier).

Here I am, twelve years later, and my breathing has become so bad that I couldn't even carry groceries up to my second floor apartment without feeling like I was going to pass out when I got to the top. So, I made a doctor's appointment. I wanted to find out what was going on. This was in October 2006. My doctor sent me for an x-ray and a pulmonary function test. When those results came back he said there was definitely a problem, so he sent me to see a lung specialist.

This doctor sent me for a CT scan and a different pulmonary function test. So, I got these results back and they showed a definite problem. This doctor recommended a bronchoscopy so they could get a biopsy. The only problem was he couldn't do it because he was crippled with arthritis and he told me I would need to find another lung doctor to perform the procedure. I found another lung specialist and he agreed that the bronchoscopy needed to be done. That was done in December 2006. They were unable to make a determination from this procedure.

Next, he talked to me about doing another open lung biopsy. I was terrified. There was no way that I wanted to go through that again. I just knew I couldn't do it.

I went to see a surgeon about doing the operation. Because of my previous surgery, he really didn't want to go in on the same side because of complications the scar tissue could cause. He sent me for more tests to see if the left lung was as bad as the right. When these tests came back they revealed that my right lung was receiving no blood flow at all. After many more tests and procedures, they finally re-diagnosed me with fibrosing mediastinitis. Because of this disease I also have severe pulmonary hypertension.

This fibrosis is a scar tissue that has wrapped itself around my arteries and veins squeezing them off. Because of this scar tissue I am not a candidate for a lung transplant.

My right pulmonary artery is completely blocked so they tried to go in and stent it, but were unsuccessful. I found out also that the left pulmonary vein was almost completely blocked. The doctors were giving me just months to live if they couldn't put a stent in the vein. I had to see a pediatric cardiologist because he was used to working with small veins. The stent was placed and appeared to return blood flow through the vein. For the first few days afterward, things seemed pretty good. After that, everything started going downhill. I started having excruciating pain in my chest and problems with my breathing.

This disease has progressed so fast over the last year that I am on oxygen 24/7 now and it seems I can't stay out of the hospital for more than a few weeks at a time. In July, I had a three week stay in the hospital. I went because I couldn't breathe, my oxygen levels kept dropping and I couldn't get them to stay up. While in the hospital I started coughing up blood and lots of it. They had to do an emergency surgery to the right lung. It was called an embolization (closing off the blood vessels). The doctor never expected me to make it home from the hospital that time. I am still dealing with this and many more symptoms.

I have been in the hospital at least 8 to 10 times since March 2007 and most of my stays have been long. I do not believe that I could have made it through any of this without my family right there by my side. The love and encouragement that they have shown is truly beyond human understanding. To be a part of God's family is a blessing.

In the last year my life has been turned upside down and inside out. I have learned to love and to be loved!

The pictures and videos on this website are so very precious to me because they are about the love of God. God has touched so many people through my illness. I am thankful that he chose to use me.

Sheila lost her battle with FM on November 15th, 2011.

David M

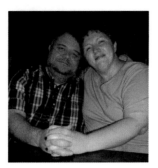

David was born in Fairfield, California, but raised in Louisiana. He spent three years in Bossier City, Louisiana and then in Winnfield until he was twenty years old.

"There was a black bird epidemic in Bossier when we lived there and although I was not school age, my older siblings were. While the epidemic was going on they had to wear their rain coats going to and from the bus stop to keep bird droppings off their clothes." (In 1976, an article was written about several incidences of high populations of blackbirds in certain areas from the late 1940s to the mid-1970s that are believed to be related to epidemics of histoplasmosis.)[xxxiii]

David began to have shortness of breath, extreme fatigue, chest pain, and hemoptysis.

"Before I was diagnosed with FM I was dealing with many symptoms. Every time I would go to the doctor they would just say I needed to lose a few pounds and I would feel better. It was not until I started coughing up large amounts of blood, at the age of twenty seven, did they begin to dig deeper to see what was causing the problem."

In 1995, David went to Schumpert Hospital in Shreveport, Louisiana where, after multiple tests (X-rays, CT scan, bronchoscopy, and an angiogram) doctors finally did a thoracotomy to get a tissue sample.

"I flat-lined twice on the operating table and then spent seventeen days in the surgical intensive care unit (SICU)."

The sample was sent Vanderbilt Hospital and David was diagnosed with post-histo FM in January 1995. His left pulmonary artery, left bronchus, and left bronchial tubes are occluded.

"After my diagnosis, I was given five years to live. I tried to go on with life as best I could and deal with the problems. Every doctor that saw me really didn't know what to do so they would just put me on prednisone and try to downplay the problem. They also gave me asthma inhalers. I believe they did this because they didn't know about the disease and didn't take time to research. I have dealt with depression, not knowing if my next flare-up would be the one that killed me."

In 2006, a stent was placed in David's left pulmonary artery in hopes that it would open the 90% blockage. It only opened it three percent. Today, David's pulmonary artery is 100% blocked with scar tissue.

"I went from working a 45-55 hour work week as a retail manager for Wal-Mart and now am totally disabled since April 2011. My wife drives me to my doctors' appointments. Aside from that, I am rarely able to leave the house because I give out so easily. My health has taken a downward spiral and it is hard to believe where I am now.

I have a great pulmonologist, Dr. Adam Wellikoff, at the Louisiana State University Medical Center (LSUMC) in Shreveport, Louisiana. He has been most caring and instrumental in getting my bronchial tubes as clear as they are now."

David has taken multiple rounds of prednisone throughout the years, as well as numerous antibiotics. He uses a CPAP machine with an oxygen concentrator with 24-hour oxygen. In order to control his bronchial swelling and bleeding, David received liquid nitrogen treatments that were instilled into his bronchial tubes.

"Dr. Adam Wellikoff and Dr. Gordon Downie performed the liquid nitrogen treatment. I was told I was the sixth person in the U.S. to receive this treatment and only the third with FM. It proved to be a success in helping with the bleeding and swelling to help control my symptoms."

"I am short of breath all the time. I have frequent bronchitis and pneumonia and will pass out a lot from lack of oxygen. I have tremendous pain in my chest area all the time. I have difficulty sleeping and am exhausted all the time. I deal with depression because I was such an active person and now I am so confined."

"We don't know what tomorrow will bring, but we know that whatever it does, my wife and I will go into it fighting and praying that one day they will find a cure for this disease so that someone else doesn't have to endure a lifetime of problems."

"I have since developed Type 2 diabetes, liver disease with esophageal and abdominal *varices*, portal hypertension, gastropathy (stomach disease), diverticulitis (infection in the large intestine), COPD, CHF, sleep apnea, chronic sinusitis, kidney disease, and GERD. I had sinus problems and gastric reflux before, but it has gotten profoundly worse." It is unlikely that these other illnesses are directly related to David's fibrosing mediastinitis.

"When I was first diagnosed I was given, at best, five years to live. Now, given all of my other health problems that have happened either as a result or in addition to my FM, my prognosis is unclear. I have been told by doctors I am receiving comfort measures to keep me breathing as well as possible and free from infection."

Idiopathic Proliferative
Fibrosing Mediastinitis (IPFM)

The three people in the following section have been diagnosed with Idiopathic Proliferative FM. IPFM lacks the calcifications (calcium build-up) that define post-histo FM. It is not as clear-cut as post-histo FM. It is also not confined to the mediastinal structures and may be found in areas such as behind the kidneys (retroperitoneal), in the neck, thyroid, behind the eye and other sites. Post-Histo FM is confined to the lymph node area of the mediastinum and, according to studies at Vanderbilt, constitutes 90% of fibrosing mediastinitis cases.

Aside from the chest area, *lesions* will typically be found in other areas of the body, confirming the diagnosis of IPFM. It is important to perform blood tests in conjunction with biopsy as to not overlook a metastatic cancer or other disease process.

Death from IPFM is rare in comparison to those people who have Post-Histo FM, especially those with post-histo bilateral involvement. Generally, the fibrosis of IPFM is less invasive and obstructive.

Unlike Post-Histo FM, there have been cases of IPFM that have improved with medications such as prednisone and, in at least one case, Tamoxifen, an estrogen blocking drug that is used to inhibit the recurrence of breast cancer. [xxxiv]

Mary

Mary grew up in Burlington, Vermont. Her shortness of breath, chest pain and cough, along with edema began in her early thirties.

In September 1986, she began seeking medical attention for her symptoms. She was told she had a variety of illnesses: Asian flu, bronchitis, asthma, allergies or simply anxiety.

"I was told that it was all in my head or I was imagining it. Finally, in May 1987, I got someone's attention that this was serious. They did tests and an exploratory thoracotomy. It was then that I was diagnosed with Idiopathic FM (IPFM)"

In December 1987, Mary had an open heart pulmonary bypass surgery at Stanford Hospital in Palo Alto, California. She later had stent placements at Sutter Memorial Hospital in Sacramento, California in 1997 and again in 1999 at the University of Washington Medical Center in Seattle, Washington, near where she now lives.

"I was told I am the only one they know of with this disease," she says of the physicians who diagnosed her. "I am in the medical history books. They have no answers for me, but, they said, they will learn a lot from me."

Mary cites her biggest frustrations as "physician ignorance, insurance issues and limitations, and the lack of support from the medical community in regards to FM and its symptoms."

When asked how FM has affected her life, Mary says that she lacks stamina and still becomes short of breath even with minimal exertion. "It's difficult to differentiate between the side effects of the meds and the effects of FM."

"In the beginning, FM affected all aspects of my life: my relationships, both personally and professionally, as well as my job. I could no longer perform my duties. As time went on, I could no longer physically take care of myself and had to resort to having a care giver regularly. Of course, then the financial thing eventually catches up with you too."

"In 2004, the doctor sent me home to die with dignity. He gave me a long list of medications and told me there was nothing more they could do for me other than to help me become 'comfortable.' I then started seeking alternative modalities and blending modern medicine with holistic. In 2005, I started living a nutritional cleansing lifestyle which made a huge impact on the quality of my life."

"Since 2005, I am truly living my life to its fullest! What we feed our bodies is exactly what they become. If I have learned anything in my 25 years of dealing with this illness this is what I have learned: I am worthy of feeling great and fully living life!"

Jeanieann

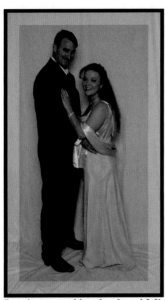

Jeanieann and her husband Michael

Jeanieann was born in Georgia and raised in South Carolina. She was diagnosed in Greenville, South Carolina with Idiopathic FM (IPFM) in 2009 after she began having difficulty breathing, sharp chest pains, facial and neck swelling and bradycardia (slow heart rate).

She underwent CT scans and biopsies of her heart and lungs in order to get her diagnosis of FM-I. Doctors have told Jeanieann that there is a football-sized mass between her lungs that extends behind her heart and wraps around her superior vena cava and she has bilateral pulmonary artery involvement. Because of this, doctors have given Jeanieann a poor prognosis.

"When we first heard the news about fibrosing mediastinitis, that day in June, everyone in the room cried. I didn't cry. I wasn't worried about the outcome. I was just scared for my family. I am a wife and a mother of four teenagers. It's hard to realize I may be leaving five amazing people without a mother or wife."

Doctors treated Jeanieann with two weeks of radiation treatment, an uncommon approach to FM. She also had a balloon angioplasty of her

SVC and stents placed in both pulmonary arteries. Recently, Jeanieann was also diagnosed with pulmonary fibrosis.

She still has persistent symptoms. "I have headaches and sharp pains when I breathe in. I cannot pull up or pick something off the floor. I get tired very easily and have to take naps. I move very slowly because if I do something wrong or I pull too much I get surreal chest pain. I do have times when my face has puffiness a little and it feels as if it's burning. Sometimes it feels as if my heart is having a hard time getting blood. Other times my face quits burning and my heart will beat the right pace again."

"Even my sex life is all messed up. I mean, a girl needs that time and I can't breathe fast enough or I have pain and I feel as if my heart is going to stop! Sorry, but it is the truth."

Jeanieann is unable to do the job she did as a special officer for a domestic violence unit. "I can't run anymore nor can I take down men and woman who are bigger than me."

Jeannieann's faith keeps her going "I am a full believer in the Son Jesus and His Father God," Jeanieann says. "Everything happens for a reason. I started a website many weeks after the news. I have studied this disease so much that I tell my doctors what they need to do. I may not be reading a book, but I am building a case and I will be going to Congress, not just for me, but for my children's children, my family and most of all, my FM family."

"I am One Person, One Voice, One Mission, I will make a Difference!"

Jeanieann invites you to visit her website at
http://fibrosingmediastinitis.webs.com/

Mary Catherine

Mary Catherine began having right-sided chest pain with worsening dyspnea and underwent a number of investigations, including CT pulmonary angiogram, MRI of the chest, and a mediastinoscopy. The growth of inflammatory and fibrotic tissue in the mediastinum led to compression and near-complete occlusion of her right pulmonary artery, resulting in symptoms of right chest pain and exertional dyspnea.

Although Mary's symptoms improved over the course of several months on systemic corticosteroid therapy, her exercise tolerance remained compromised and she required narcotic analgesics.

Mary presented initially in early 2007 with symptoms of palpitations and exertional dyspnea. Although pulmonary function tests showed evidence of airflow obstruction, her dyspnea worsened in spite of inhaled corticosteroid and bronchodilator therapy.

In mid-March 2007, Mary developed pleuritic pain in the right lower chest and back, associated with worsening dyspnea, productive cough, intermittent low grade fever, and ultimately, hemoptysis. She was treated with antibiotics for presumed pneumonia, but showed no improvement.

Chest x-rays showed a peripherally situated relatively uniform, but ill-defined spot in the right lung, consistent with a pulmonary infarct. Because of suspicion of pulmonary embolism and infarction, Mary underwent a CT pulmonary angiography on March 23, 2007, and was found to have a near complete obstruction of the right pulmonary artery, with only a trickle of blood flow. There was a soft tissue density in the right mediastinum, surrounding the right main pulmonary artery, associated with lymphadenopathy. The largest node, in the subcarinal area, measured 1.9 cm in maximal diameter. None of the nodes showed calcification. CT images confirmed a lesion consistent with infarction.

Mary was admitted to the hospital that day for further investigation and management. Physical examination did not show peripheral lymphadenopathy or hepatosplenomegaly (*enlargement of the liver and spleen*). ECG showed sinus tachycardia, without blood pressure problems. Despite the marked reduction in right lung perfusion seen on CT angiography, gas exchange was adequate. Echocardiography did not show evidence of right heart strain or thrombus within the right-sided chambers of the heart.

With anticoagulation, Mary's dyspnea and chest pain improved, and the hemoptysis subsided. She was discharged several days later with arrangements for further investigation on an outpatient basis. Based on the CT scan findings, the differential diagnosis included endobronchial malignancy with mediastinal involvement, lymphoma, fibrosing mediastinitis, and possibly an isolated pulmonary vasculitis with in-situ thrombosis of the right pulmonary artery.

Mary had subsequent investigations, including a bronchoscopy and mediastinoscopy. No endobronchial lesion was identified. The lymph nodes with the mediastinoscopy were noted to be firm and the surrounding tissue fibrotic. Multiple lymph node biopsies were taken and none showed evidence of lymphoma or other malignancy.

An MRI of the thorax confirmed soft tissue proliferation and lymphadenopathy in the right mediastinum with an appearance that was more likely inflammation than malignancy.

A perfusion lung scan was performed to quantify pulmonary perfusion on the right side. Baseline perfusion was markedly reduced.

Pulmonary function tests showed mixed restriction and obstruction with reduced diffusing capacity.

Blood tests showed no evidence of vasculitis. Histoplasmosis studies, including fungal stains of the lymph node tissue obtained with the mediastinoscopy were negative. Histoplasmosis complement fixation titers were also negative.

At the completion of these investigations, it appeared that the most likely diagnosis was fibrosing mediastinitis. In the absence of calcification of the lymph nodes, and with negative fungal stains and histoplasmosis titers it was further presumed that the fibrosing mediastinitis was idiopathic in nature, rather than post-histoplasmosis. A course of systemic corticosteroid therapy was initiated in mid-May 2007.

CT scans were repeated in June and September 2007, and showed reduction in the mediastinal inflammation and lymph node tissue. Perfusion lung scans in July 2007 and January 2008, showed no significant improvement in right lung perfusion, but repeat pulmonary function tests in November 2007, showed improvement.

Mary's condition has not changed over the past few years. She lives with her husband in London, Ontario, Canada.

A Tribute to Sheila Durham

By Mark Dalton Thompson

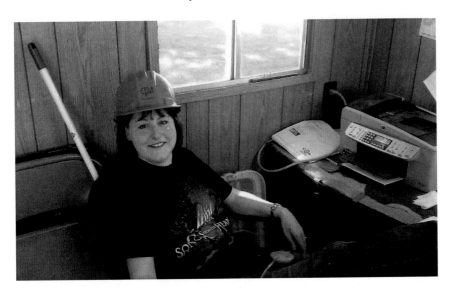

Our relationship defies all earthly logic, so I will not attempt to explain it. As her sister Cathy ("Awesome Angel") once said, "It speaks for itself. Anyone can feel the love that you two share."

When I met Sheila, she was in the lobby of her Group Home where we were working on a major renovation project. She was sitting in her scooter with a pink house robe, no makeup, and oxygen in her nose. She was beautiful. There was an undeniable spiritual presence that flowed from her.

We arranged to have dinner and, later, we went to Bass Pro. It was during our day at Bass Pro that I became aware of the awesome burden that FM brought to her. It was also the day that she allowed me to become her caregiver.

My duties involved loading her accessible van, exchanging oxygen tanks, and monitoring her oxygen saturation. I also assisted her with brief periods of very slow walking. I was educated to the life limiting effects that FM had placed upon her.

At the same time though, I was amazed at the fullness of her spirit and joy of precious life.

At the time, I was extremely self-absorbed and arrogant. I just knew that I could teach her so much about living on earth and preparing for what would come afterwards. I termed it "Angel Training." I should have known from the look in her eyes that it was I who would be trained.

It was the first time in my life that I actually felt the desire to do EVERYTHING possible to make someone else's life better. I learned the minute to minute challenges of living a life where a walk to the bathroom for her was the equivalent of my running a mile. The fluctuations in her oxygen levels and my ability to anticipate and recognize those effects and jump to immediate action to remedy those effects were, at a minimum, shocking.

The primary method that we used to improve her oxygen levels was the rhythmic application of hand blows to her back.* When she awoke from sleeping, her mediastinum would be congested with a fluid mass that was not unlike concrete mix. I learned to feel and listen, from the back blows, the worst points of congestion and how to directionally apply the blows to break up the fluid while waiting for the medication to push the fluids from her body. Sheila had no right lung function. Surgical stents had been placed, but she had 30% pulmonary capacity at best.

My education involved staying awake as she slept, listening to her struggled respiration. I would gently move her to better position while monitoring her oxygen saturation without awakening her.

Different foods had a great impact upon the degree of fluid accumulation. Her primary sustenance would be fruits and raw vegetables. She loved stuff that was bad for her, but, as her physician, Dr. Ramirez said, "Things that bring joy into a life of any condition should not be totally avoided." Sheila was addicted to excellent guacamole and chips. So was I.

Sheila was hospitalized four times during the nine months that we were together. Each time it was brought about by a combination of over exertion and exposure to another person's contagious condition.

Her one year-old granddaughter, Naomi, was the most precious element in her life, closely followed by her daughter

Kayla. Sheila obsessively doted upon and mentored their lives. No one ever loved their child and grandchild more. Her sister, Cathy Bailey, provided unfailing care and support to Sheila. We called her "Awesome Angel." She is all that. Also, Melissa May "Missie," was her very best Friend. Missie is family to me and a giver of God's Love. Sheila could not resist holding Naomi, whom we called "Nomers," close even when she was ill.

During Sheila's third hospitalization she coded three times with oxygen levels dropping into the sixties. The staff at Audubon [Louisville] did a miraculous job with her care. They all knew Sheila. It was not just me that felt the strong presence of God within her.

I was on the way to a project in Nebraska when I visited Sheila on what would be her last night. She was in critical care with a CPAP and 15 liters oxygen. I fed her the last meal she would eat. She was still "bossing" me and the staff, not as to her needs, but as to what we should be doing to take care of ourselves.

I called her friend Kim to ask that she stay with Sheila that night. I am forever grateful that she did. As Sheila slept, I kissed her goodbye and departed.

She passed at 4 a.m. on November 15th, 2011. She was 37 years old.

Kim told me that just before she died, Sheila sat up glowingly, smiled and reached out with both arms. God took her peacefully.

Yes, indeed. "Angel Training."

*Author's Note: see postural drainage in the glossary

Glossary

Angiogram (Angiography): \'an-jē-ə-ˌgram\ An interventional radiologist performs this X-ray procedure, which is also called an angiogram. During the angiogram, the doctor inserts a thin tube (catheter) into the artery through a small nick in the skin about the size of the tip of a pencil. A substance called a contrast agent (X-ray dye) is injected to make the blood vessels visible on the X-ray.

One of the most common reasons for angiograms is to see if there is a blockage or narrowing in a blood vessel that may interfere with the normal flow of blood through the body. In many cases, the interventional radiologist can treat a blocked blood vessel without surgery at the same time the angiogram is performed. Interventional radiologists treat blockages with techniques called angioplasty and thrombolysis.

Acquired Immunity: Occurring as a result of prior exposure to an infectious agent or its antigens. We develop this by simply living in the cold cruel world.

Alveolus (plural alveoli): \al-'vē-ə-ləs\ Air sacs in the lungs where oxygen is exchanged through the bloodstream.

Amphotericin-B: \ˌam(p)-fə-'ter-ə-sən\ A potent intravenous anti-fungal that should be administered primarily to patients with progressive, potentially life-threatening fungal infections.

Antibody: A protein produced by the body's immune system when it detects harmful substances, called antigens.

Antigen: Any substance that causes your immune system to produce antibodies against it.

Artery: Larger, thicker blood vessels that carry blood away from the heart. Examples: carotid artery, femoral artery, pulmonary artery, aorta.

Asymptomatic: Having no symptoms.

Atelectasis: \ˌat-əl-ˈek-tə-səs\ Collapse of the lung, partially or completely.

Atrial Fibrillation (A-Fib): An abnormal heart rhythm that causes the heart's two upper chambers, called the atria, to contract very fast and irregularly.

Bronchoalveolar \ˌbräŋ-kō-al-ˈvē-ə-lər\ Lavage (BAL): procedure for collecting the cellular material of the alveoli (microorganisms, types of inflammatory cells) by use of a bronchoscope or other hollow tube through which saline is instilled into distal bronchi and then withdrawn.

Bronchoscopy: A procedure performed with an endoscope in order to inspect the airways of the lung.

Bronchus: (plural bronchi, adjective bronchial) is a passage of airway in the respiratory tract that conducts air into the lungs. The bronchus branches into smaller tubes, which in turn become bronchioles.

Calcification: A build-up of calcium salts in soft tissue that cause hardening.

Carina: \kə-ˈrī-nə, -ˈrē-\ The junction of the trachea where it divides into the two mainstem bronchi.

Cardiac catheterization: A procedure done to check blood flow in the coronary arteries , blood flow and blood pressure in the chambers of the heart , find out how well the heart valves work, and check for defects in the way the wall of the heart moves. It is typically done in the cardiac catheterization lab. (cath lab).

Cardiomyopathy: \KAR-de-o-mi-OP-ah-thee\ A heart disease in which the muscle of the heart becomes rigid, thickened or enlarged and leads to heart failure, heart valve damage or irregular heart rhythms.

Caseous: A form of necrosis in which tissue is changed into a dry, amorphous mass resembling cheese.

CHF: *see Congestive Heart Failure*

Chloride Sweat Test or Sweat Test: A test to determine if someone has cystic fibrosis. It should be noted that there is no connection between FM and cystic fibrosis.

Chronic Obstructive Pulmonary Disease (COPD): A lung disease, primarily caused by smoking. The two types of COPD include chronic bronchitis and emphysema which causes destruction of the lung tissue over time.

Coccidiomycosis \käk-͵sid-ē-ō-mī-ˈkō-səs\ Also known as Valley Fever. It is a fungal disease caused by *Coccidioides immitis* or *C. posadasi*. It is endemic in certain parts of Arizona, California, Nevada, New Mexico, Texas, Utah and northwestern Mexico.

COPD: *see Chronic Obstructive Pulmonary Disease*

Congestive Heart Failure (CHF): A condition in which the heart becomes an ineffective pump, causing fluid to build up in the lungs and other areas of the body. Many things may cause CHF, including underlying heart disease, heart attack, high blood pressure, infection, and some lung diseases.

Coronary Arteries: Small vessels that supply blood and oxygen to the heart muscle.

Coronary Artery Vasculitis; Inflammation of the arteries that feed the heart muscle.

Cor Pulmonale: Enlargement or failure of the right side of the heart. May be caused from long term pulmonary hypertension.

Corticosteroids: A group of natural and synthetic hormones secreted by the pituitary gland. These include glucocorticoids, which are anti-inflammatory agents with a large number of other functions; mineralocorticoids, which control salt and water balance primarily through action on the kidneys; and corticotropins, which control secretion of hormones by the pituitary gland. Also, man-made drugs used to treat inflammatory diseases. May be referred to as: Methylprednisolone (Solu-Medrol), Prednisone, Steroids. These are not the same as anabolic steroids used by some..ahem..athletes.

Coumadin (warfarin): a medication used to prevent blood clots from forming or growing larger in your blood and blood vessels. It is prescribed for people with certain types of irregular heartbeat, people with prosthetic (replacement or mechanical) heart valves, and people who have suffered a heart attack. Warfarin is also used to treat or prevent venous thrombosis (swelling and blood clot in a vein) and pulmonary embolism (a blood clot in the lung). Warfarin is in a class of medications called anticoagulants ('blood thinners'). It works by decreasing the clotting ability of the blood. Yes, it is the basis for some rat poisons, but it is not a poison, per se. It kills rats because the rats lack the ability to vomit so the warfarin causes them to die from internal bleeding.

Computerized Tomography (CT or CAT): An x-ray used to give more detail. Sometimes dye is injected into your vein in order to enhance the pictures or to visualize blood flow. (see CT angio)

CT Angiography (CT angio or CTA): Angiography involves the injection of contrast dye into a large blood vessel, usually in your leg, to help visualize the blood vessels and the blood flow within them. When the contrast dye is used to visualize your veins, the study is called a venogram, and when it is used to visualize your arteries, it is known as an arteriogram. CT angiography is similar to a CT scan, but the contrast dye is injected into one of your veins shortly before the x ray image is performed. Because the dye is injected into a vein rather than into an artery, as in traditional angiography, CT angiography could be considered less invasive.

Dysphagia: \dis-ˈfā-j(ē-)ə\ Difficulty swallowing.

Dyspnea: Shortness of breath. (see exertional dyspnea)

Ectopic: Occurring in an abnormal position or place.

Edema: Swelling of an organ or tissue.

Effusion: The escape of fluid from the blood vessels or lymphatics into the tissues or a cavity.

Esophagus: A muscular tube connecting the throat (pharynx) with the stomach. The esophagus is about 8 inches long, and is lined by moist pink tissue called mucosa.

Exertional Dyspnea: Shortness of breath with activity.

Fibrosis: The formation of excess fibrous connective tissue in an organ or tissue in a reparative or reactive process. In FM, this fibrosis is typically caused by calcifications along the lymph nodes.

Fluoroscopy: continuous image of an x-ray used during procedures to aid physicians in diagnosing and performing therapeutic measures.

Fungus (pl. fungi): A large group of organisms, including some microorganisms such as yeasts and molds. Larger fungi include mushrooms. Fungi are crucial to the fermentation process for the creation of beer and wine. Medications, such as penicillin, are derived from molds. They typically reproduce by producing spores. Some fungi produce poisonous substances called mycotoxins and may cause harm to humans and animals. The fungus itself can also be the culprit in some diseases. Fungal diseases include ringworm, athlete's foot, coccidioidomycosis (Valley Fever), and histoplasmosis.

GERD: Gastroesophageal reflux disease. Stomach contents backing up into the esophagus, causing symptoms of heartburn.

Granuloma: A small area of tissue inflammation usually caused by an infection. An accumulation of macrophages, typically found in the lungs. (adj. *granulomatous*)

Hemoptysis: Coughing up blood.

Histoplasmosis: A fungal disease caused by the Histoplasmosis capitulatum primarily affecting the lungs.

Host: In biology, the organism that harbors an invader.

Human Leukocyte Antigen (HLA): A group of protein molecules located on bone marrow cells that can provoke an immune response. (self-producing antigens).

Idiopathic: arising spontaneously or from an obscure or unknown cause.

Immune Response: (inflammatory response or inflammation) occurs when tissues are injured by bacteria, trauma, toxins, heat, or any other cause. The damaged cells release chemicals that cause blood vessels to leak fluid into the tissues, causing swelling. This helps isolate the foreign substance from further contact with body tissues.

Immunocompromised: A state of weakened or absent immune system. May be caused by genetics, HIV, certain cancers, including leukemia, lymphoma, or multiple myeloma, corticosteroid use, chemotherapy, radiation, immunosuppressive post-transplant medications, or pregnancy.

Infarction: Death of tissue due to shutting off the blood supply. (Myocardial infarction AKA MI is a heart attack)

Innate Immunity: First line of defense against disease, includes skin, mucus membranes, the ability to cough and sneeze, and the body's immune response.

INR: International Normalized Ratio. A standard of measurement for protime, or how quickly blood clots. A normal INR is 1. For people receiving anticoagulants, such as Coumadin (warfarin) the INR ranges from 2.0 to 4.0.

Intubation: A long plastic tube, called an endotracheal tube, is placed into the airway to assist with breathing.

Ischemia: A decrease in blood supply to an organ or tissue caused from obstruction or constriction of blood vessels.

Itraconazole: Brand name: Sporanox. Medication used to treat fungal infections. Potentially helpful for acute histoplasmosis infections, but not found to be helpful in patients already diagnosed with fibrosing mediastinitis. Also extremely expensive.

Lesion Any localized, abnormal structural change in the body.

Lymph: A clear, watery fluid that acts to remove bacteria and certain proteins from the tissues, transport fat from the small intestine, and supply mature lymphocytes to the blood.

Lymphadenopathy: A chronic, abnormal enlargement of the lymph nodes, usually associated with disease.

Lymph node: Any of the small, bean-shaped structures, located along the lymphatic vessels, which supply lymphocytes to the bloodstream and remove bacteria and foreign particles from the lymph.

Lymphocyte: Any of the nearly colorless cells formed in lymphoid tissue, as in the lymph nodes, spleen, thymus, and tonsils, constituting between 22 and 28 percent of all white blood cells in the blood of a normal adult human. They function in the development of immunity and include two specific types, B cells and T cells.

Macrophage: A type of white blood cell that "eats" foreign matter.

Mediastinoscopy: a surgical procedure in which a tube (a mediastinoscope) is inserted through the chest wall to examine the area between the lungs (the mediastinum). Biopsies of tissue can be obtained for diagnosis.

Mediastinum: It contains the heart, the great vessels of the heart, the esophagus, the trachea, the phrenic nerve, the cardiac nerve, the thoracic duct, the thymus, and the lymph nodes of the central chest.

Methacholine Challenge: a test used to diagnose asthma. Also called bronchial challenge test.

Myocardial infarction (MI): A heart attack. Caused by an interruption in blood flow to the heart muscle due to blockage of one or more of the coronary arteries.

Myocardium: The muscle of the heart.

Odynophagia: \ō-ˌdin-ə-ˈfā-j(ē-)ə\ Painful swallowing

Oxygen saturation (O2 sat): A measure of how much oxygen the blood is carrying as a percentage of the maximum it could carry. Measured with a device called a pulse oximeter or pulse ox. It is affixed to the fingertip and detects oxygen saturation through the nail beds. Ideally 92-99%.

Pericardium: The fluid filled sac that surrounds the heart and the proximal ends of the aorta, vena cava, and the pulmonary artery. (adj: pericardial)

PICC: peripherally inserted central catheter. It is long, slender, small, flexible tube that is inserted into a peripheral vein, typically in the upper arm, and advanced until the catheter tip terminates in a large vein in the chest near the heart to obtain intravenous access.

Pleura: The membrane around the lungs. When it becomes inflamed it is referred to as pleurisy. (Pleuritic: pertaining to the pleura)

Pneumonectomy: A surgical procedure to remove a lung. The removal of part of the lung is called a lobectomy.

Pneumonia: An inflammation of the lungs, especially affecting the alveoli.

Portal System: Veins that drain blood from the abdominal organs of the digestive tract, spleen, gallbladder, and pancreas and transferred to the liver through the portal vein. Increased blood pressure in this area is called *portal hypertension* and is caused when blood vessels in the liver are blocked.

Positive End-Expiratory Pressure (PEEP): A method of mechanical ventilation in which pressure is maintained to keep the alveoli from completely collapsing on exhale. This helps improve oxygen and carbon dioxide exchange.

Prednisone: Prednisone is in a class of medications called corticosteroids. It works to treat patients with low levels of corticosteroids by replacing steroids that are normally produced naturally by the body. It works to treat other conditions by reducing swelling and redness and by changing the way the immune system works. *(see Corticosteroids)*

Prothrombin time. (PT or protime) Measures how quickly blood clots. (see INR)

PTFE (Polytetrafluoroethylene) Graft : A Teflon graft used to bypass stenosed vessels when a donor vessel is not suitable or available.

Pulmonary artery catheter (PA Catheter): flow-directed balloon-tipped pulmonary artery catheter (PAC) (also known as the Swan-Ganz or right heart catheter). It is inserted percutaneously (through the skin) into a major vein (jugular, subclavian, femoral) via an introducer sheath.

Pulmonary embolism (PE): The sudden blockage of a major blood vessel (artery) in the lung, usually by a blood clot. Most common symptoms include: Sudden shortness of breath, sharp chest pain that is worse when you cough or take a deep breath, and a cough that brings up pink, foamy mucus.

Pulmonary Hypertension: Abnormally high blood pressure in the arteries of the lungs, putting strain on the right heart and making it work harder than normal.

Resection: Surgical removal of part of an organ or a structure.

Right middle lobe syndrome (RMLS): The collapse (atelectasis) of the right middle lobe of the lung. Can be seen in young people with asthma, but no absolute clinical definition.

Sarcoidosis: A disease in which inflammation occurs in the lymph nodes, lungs, liver, eyes, skin, or other tissues.

Stenosis: A narrowing of a structure.

Stent: a small mesh tube that's used to treat narrow or weak blood vessels, especially arteries. They have also been used in veins. The term stent may also refer to any type of medical device used to treat narrowing of an anatomic structure.

Sternum: The breastbone.

Superior Vena Cava Syndrome (SVC Syndrome): A blockage of the second largest vein in the body. Symptoms include: Swelling around the eye, swelling of the face, or swelling of the whites of the eyes. The most common symptoms are shortness of breath (dyspnea) and swelling of the face, neck, trunk, and arms. *(see Vena Cava)*

Syncope: Temporary loss of consciousness or fainting, usually occurring when there is drop in blood flow to the brain.

Tissue plasminogen activator: (abbreviated tPA or PLAT) is a protein involved in the breakdown of blood clots. It is used to dissolve blood clots in stroke and other clotting conditions. Its use is controversial. It can cause severe bleeding.

Thoracotomy: A surgical opening of the chest wall.

Thrombosis: A blood clot formed inside a blood vessel.

Thymus: The thymus produces types of white blood cells called "T-lymphocytes," which help fight infection. This gland functions primarily in infancy and childhood to help build up the immune system. After puberty, the thymus gradually shrinks, reaching only about 15% of its maximum size by middle age.

tPA: *(see Tissue plasminogen activator)*

Trachea: the windpipe, the tube that connects the nose and mouth to the lungs.

Varices: A type of varicose vein that develops in the lining of the esophagus and the stomach in certain diseases, such as liver disease. Caused by pressure that builds up in a large vein in the liver (portal vein).

Vein: Thinner walled blood vessels that carry blood back to the heart. Examples: superior vena cava, internal jugular vein

Vena Cava: The superior vena cava (SVC) is the large vein which returns blood to the heart from the head, neck and both upper limbs. The inferior vena cava (IVC) returns blood to the heart from the lower part of the body.

Ventilation/Perfusion Scan (V/Q or Lung scan): A test performed by a nuclear medicine technician where the lung's ability to capture air is assessed by using a radioactive isotope mist (ventilation). Then a radioisotope is injected into the bloodstream to assess blood flow through the lungs. (Perfusion scan).

Vertigo: A form of dizziness that makes the room feel like it is moving.

Medical Facilities and Physicians

These physicians and facilities are mentioned in DERAILED. This is by no means a comprehensive list of caregivers, nor do they specifically specialize in patients with fibrosing mediastinitis.

CALIFORNIA

Stanford University Medical Center
300 Pasteur Drive
Palo Alto, CA 94304
(650) 723-4000
http://stanfordhospital.org/

Sutter Memorial Hospital
5151 F Street
Sacramento, CA 95819
916-454-3333
http://www.suttermedicalcenter.org/

University of California San Diego Health Systems (UCSD)
200 West Arbor Dr.
San Diego, CA 92103
858-657-7000
http://health.ucsd.edu

Kim M. Kerr, M.D.
Professor of Clinical Medicine
Director, Medical Intensive Care Unit - Thornton
UC San Diego Division of Pulmonary & Critical Care Medicine
9300 Campus Point Drive, #7381
La Jolla, CA 92037-7381
To schedule an appointment with Dr. Kerr, contact Sue Brick at 858-657-7132

GEORGIA

Georgia Health Sciences Medical Center
1120 15th Street
Augusta, GA 30912
(706) 721-CARE (2273)
800-736-CARE (2273)
http://www.mcghealth.org

ILLINOIS

Sandra L Ettema, MD
Otolaryngology
301 N 8th St
Rm 5B
Springfield, IL 62701

Mark R Johnson, MD SIU Clinics
Pediatric pulmonology
301 N 8th St Rm 3A169
Springfield, IL

Memorial Medical Center
701 North First Street
Springfield, Illinois 62781
 (217) 788-3000
https://www.memorialmedical.com/

INDIANA

IU Health University Hospital
550 University Blvd.
 Indianapolis, IN 46202
(317) 944-5000
http://iuhealth.org

Lutheran Hospital Ft. Wayne
7950 W Jefferson Blvd.
Fort Wayne, IN 46804
(800) 444-2001

http://www.lutheranhospital.com/

IOWA

University of Iowa Hospitals and Clinics
200 Hawkins Drive
Iowa City, IA 52242
Local Phone: 319-356-1616
Toll Free: 800-777-8442
http://www.uihealthcare.org/

KENTUCKY

Norton Audubon Hospital
1 Audubon Plaza Drive
Louisville, KY 40217
(888) 4-U-NORTON / (888) 486-6786
http://www.nortonhealthcare.com/nortonaudubonhospital

LOUISIANA

CHRISTUS Highland Medical Center
1453 E. Bert Kouns Industrial Loop
Shreveport, Louisiana
318.681.5000
http://www.christusschumpert.org

Louisiana State University Medical Center   (LSUMC)

1501 Kings Highway
P.O. Box 33932
Shreveport, LA 71130-3932
(318)675.5000
http://lsuhscshreveport.edu/lsumedicalcenter

MICHIGAN

University of Michigan Health Systems
1500 East Medical Center Drive
Ann Arbor, MI 48109
(734) 936-4000
http://www.med.umich.edu/

MINNESOTA

Mayo Clinic
200 1st St SW # W4
Rochester, MN 55905
Mayo Clinic in Minnesota
507-538-3270
7 a.m. to 6 p.m. Central time, Monday through
Friday
http://www.mayoclinic.com/

MISSOURI

Barnes Jewish Hospital
One Barnes-Jewish Hospital Plaza
St. Louis, MO 63110
(866) 867-3627 or (866) TOP-DOCS
http://www.barnesjewish.org/

St. Louis Children's Hospital
One Children's Place
St. Louis, MO 63110
314.454.6000
http://www.stlouischildrens.org

NEVADA

Children's Heart Center
3006 South Maryland Parkway
Suite 690
Las Vegas, NV 89109

Telephone: Las Vegas (702) 732-1290 or Toll Free: (866) 732-1290
E-mail: info@childrensheartcenter.com
http://www.childrensheartcenter.com

Abraham Rothman, M. D.
Pediatric Cardiology
Children's Heart Center, Las Vegas Nevada

NORTH CAROLINA

Duke University Hospital
2301 Erwin Road
Durham, NC 27710
888-ASK-DUKE (888-275-3853)
http://www.dukehealth.org/

OHIO

Bethesda North Hospital
10500 Montgomery Road
Cincinnati, OH 45242-4402
(513) 865-1111
http://www.trihealth.com/hospitals-and-practices/bethesda-north-hospital/

Cleveland Clinic
9500 Euclid Avenue
Cleveland, OH 44195
866.320.4573
http://my.clevelandclinic.org

The Ohio State University
410 W. 10th Ave.
Columbus, OH 43210
614-293-8000
http://medicalcenter.osu.edu

Nationwide Children's Hospital
700 Children's Drive
Columbus, Ohio 43205
(614)722-2000
http://www.nationwidechildrens.org/

PENNSYLVANIA
Thomas Jefferson University Hospitals
111 South 11th Street
Philadelphia, PA 19107
215-955-6000
http://www.jeffersonhospital.org/

TENNESSEE

Baptist Memorial
Baptist Memorial Hospital-Memphis
6019 Walnut Grove Rd.
Memphis, TN 38120
901-226-5000
info.memphis@bmhcc.org
http://www.baptistonline.org/memphis/

James E. Loyd, M.D.
Medicine: Allergy, Pulmonary, and Critical Care
Rudy W. Jacobson Professor of Medicine,VICC
Member
Researcher
Vanderbilt University Medical Center
C1208, MCN
1161 21st Ave.
Nashville, TN 37232-2650
615-322-3412

Thomas P. Doyle, M.D.
Division of Cardiology
2200 Children's Way
5230 Doctors' Office Tower
Nashville, TN 37232-9119

Phone: (615) 322-7447
Fax: (615) 322-2210

Vanderbilt University Medical Center
1211 Medical Center Drive
Nashville, TN 37232
(615) 322-5000
http://www.vanderbilthealth.com/main/

TEXAS

Texas Heart Institute
6770 Bertner Avenue
Houston, Texas 77030
(832)355-4011
http://www.texasheartinstitute.org/

WASHINGTON

University of Washington Medical Center
1959 N.E. Pacific St.
Seattle, WA 98195
General Information: 206.598.3300
http://www.uwmedicine.org/patient-
care/locations/uwmc/Pages/default.aspx

WISCONSIN

Bellin Health Systems
744 South Webster Avenue
 P.O. Box 23400
 Green Bay, WI 54305-3400
(920) 433-3500
http://bellin.org/

Marshfield Clinic - Marshfield Center
1000 North Oak Avenue
Marshfield, WI 54449
715-387-5511 or 1-800-782-8581
http://www.marshfieldclinic.org

North Shore Medical Center
Ministry Door County Medical Center
323 South 18th Avenue
Sturgeon Bay, WI 54235-1495
(920)743-5566
(800)522-8919
http://ministryhealth.org/

CANADA
St. Joseph's Health Care Hamilton
Charlton Campus
50 Charlton Avenue East, Hamilton, Ontario,
Canada L8N   4A6
(905) 522 - 1155 (automated)
(905) 522 - 4941 (switchboard)
http://www.stjosham.on.ca/

Research and Resources

The author does not endorse or recommend any commercial products, processes, or services mentioned. The views and opinions of contributors expressed in DERAILED does not necessarily state or reflect those of the author.

Some Web pages may provide links to other Internet sites for the convenience of users. The author is not responsible for the availability or content of these external sites, nor does the author endorse, warrant, or guarantee the products, services, or information described or offered at these other Internet sites.

WEBSITES

Fibrosing Mediastinitis Informational Website
Email: tlewy1@yahoo.com
http://www.fibrosing-mediastinitis.com

Living with FM
http://livingwithfm.org
Information and resources for people with FM

Twitter
http://twitter.com/ourfmlife

My FM Life
http://myfmlife.com
The author's personal page

FM Patient Community Group
http://rarediseases.bensfriends.org/group/fibrosing-mediastinitis

Fibrosing Mediastinitis and More
Rick's site
http://fibrosingmediastinitisandmore.com/

Facebook Group for People with FM
http://www.facebook.com/groups/fibrosingmediastini
tis/

Our Walk on the Path of Fibrosing Mediastinitis
Jeanieann's Site
http://fibrosingmediastinitis.webs.com/

**National Organization for Rare Disorders
(NORD)**
http://www.rarediseases.org/rare-disease-
information/rare-diseases/byID/1177/viewAbstract

Pulmonary Hypertension Association
http://www.phassociation.org/

**Genetic and Rare Diseases Information Center
(GARD)**
http://rarediseases.info.nih.gov/GARD/Condition/833
7/Fibrosing_mediastinitis.aspx

Mediastinal Fibrosis
Cody's Site
http://mediastinalfibrosis.webs.com/

The FM Foundation
http://www.thefmfoundation.org/

Healthaplenty Isagenix Independent Associate
Mary Burrell
http://healthaplenty.isagenix.com/us/en/company_ass
ociate.dhtml

BOOKS

Askren, TJ. Derailed: Living with Fibrosing Mediastinitis (2012)

Chodron, Pema. The Places that Scare You: A Guide to Fearlessness in Difficult Times. Shambhala. (August 13, 2002).

Chodron, Pema. When Things Fall Apart: Heart Advice for Difficult Times. Shambhala. 2000.

Ongoing Research

James Loyd, M.D., Professor of Medicine, Division of Allergy, Pulmonary & Critical Care at Vanderbilt University School of Medicine in Nashville, Tennessee, is conducting a study of fibrosing mediastinitis, using persons with fibrosing mediastinitis who voluntarily submit their medical test results. For more information, please contact:

James E. Loyd, MD
Vanderbilt University Medical Center
Nashville, TN 37232-2650
615-322-3412
jim.loyd@vanderbilt.edu

Information on current clinical trials is posted on the Internet at www.clinicaltrials.gov. All studies receiving U.S. government funding, and some supported by private industry, are posted on this government web site.

For information about clinical trials being conducted at the NIH Clinical Center in Bethesda, MD, contact the NIH Patient Recruitment Office:

Tollfree: (800) 411-1222
TTY: (866) 411-1010
Email: prpl@cc.nih.gov

References

[i] Goodwin RA, Nickell JA, Des Prez RM. Mediastinal fibrosis complicating healed primary histoplasmosis and tuberculosis. Medicine (Baltimore). 1972;51(3):227.

[ii] Meredith E. Pugh, MD; and James E. Loyd, MD. Fibrosing Mediastinitis: Causes, Diagnosis, and Treatment. PCCSU Article | 01.15.09.

[iii] Loyd JE, Tillman BF, Atkinson JB, Des Prez RM. Mediastinal fibrosis complicating histoplasmosis. Medicine (Baltimore) 1988; 67:295.

[v] Wheat LJ, Kohler RB, Tewari RP. Diagnosis of disseminated histoplasmosis by detection of Histoplasma capsulatum antigen in serum and urine specimens. N Engl J Med. 1986 Jan 9;314(2):83-8.

[ ] Wheat LJ., Slama TG, Eitzen HE, et al. A large urban outbreak of histoplasmosis: clinical features. Ann Intern Med 1981; 94:331.

[vi] Lihteh, Wu, et.al. Presumed Ocular Histoplasmosis Syndrome. http://www.emedicine.com/oph/topic406.htm. 07/24/2007.

[vii] Rozenblit AM, Kim A, Tuvia J, Wenig BM. Adrenal histoplasmosis manifested as Addison's disease: unusual CT features with magnetic resonance imaging correlation. Clin Radiol. 2001 Aug;56(8):682-4.

[viii] Tai YF, Kullmann DM, Howard RS, Scott GM, Hirsch NP, Revesz T, Leary SM. Central nervous system histoplasmosis in an immunocompetent patient. J Neurol. 2010 Nov; 257(11):1931-3. Epub 2010 Jun 22.

[ ] Rosenthal, J. Rheumatologic manifestations of histoplasmosis in the recent Indianapolis epidemic. Arthritis & Rheumatism. Volume 26, Issue 9. September 1983.1065–1070.
Wheat, LJ. 1986.
[ ] Snm.org. Society of Nuclear Medicine and Molecular Imaging. 2012.
[i] http://www.medicinenet.com/mri_scan/article.htm#1whatis
[ii] http://www.nhlbi.nih.gov/health/health-topics/topics/bron/during.html
[v] http://www.hopkinsmedicine.org/healthlibrary/test_procedures/pulmonary mediastinoscopy_92,P07753/
[ ] Wheat LJ. Histoplasmosis susceptibility in humans. In: Fungal Disease, Jacobs H, Nall L (Eds), Marcel Dekker, New York 1997. P. 239.

[xvi] Chu JH, Feudtner C, Heydon K, et al. Hospitalizations for endemic mycoses: a population-based national study. Clin Infect Dis 2006; 42;822.

[xvii] Lucille Enix and Tricia Edgell. The FM Report. 2007.

[xviii] Interview with Dr. James Loyd. Rudy W. Jacobson , Professor of Medicine, Vanderbilt University Medical Center, Nashville, Tennessee. July, 2003.

[xix] Hage CA, Ribes JA, Wengenack NL, et al. A multicenter evaluation of tests for diagnosis of histoplasmosis. Clin Infect Dis 2011; 53:448.

[xx] H. Edward Garrett, Jr., M.D., Charles L. Roper, M.D. Surgical Intervention in Histoplasmosis. Division of Cardiothoracic Surgery, Washington University School of Medicine, St. Louis, MO. Ann Thorac Surg 1986;42:711-722.

[xxi] Loyd, et al. 1988.

[xxii] Gustafson MR, Moulton MJ. Fibrosing mediastinitis with severe bilateral pulmonary artery narrowing: RV-RPA bypass with a homograft conduit Tex Heart Inst J. 2012;39(3):412-5.

[xxiii] Loyd, et al.

[xxiv] Christopher J. Smolock, MD, Shanda Blackmon, MD. Journal of Vascular Surgery Volume 56, Issue 2 , Pages 492-495, August 2012

[xxv] Wheat LJ., Slama TG, Eitzen HE, et al. A large urban outbreak of histoplasmosis: clinical features. Ann Intern Med 1981; 94:331.

[xxvi] H. Edward Garrett, Jr., M.D., Charles L. Roper, M.D. Surgical Intervention in Histoplasmosis. Ann Thorac Surg 1986;42:711-722.

[xxvii] de Mello-Filho FV, Antonio SM, Carrau RL
Endoscopically placed expandable metal tracheal stents for the management of complicated tracheal stenosis. Am J Otolaryngol. 2003 Jan-Feb;24(1):34-40.
.

[xxviii] Kalra M, Gloviczki P, Andrews JC, et al. Open surgical and endovascular treatment of superior vena cava syndrome caused by nonmalignant disease. J Vasc Surg 2003; 38:215.

[xxix] Alazemi,,Saleh S. Lunn ,William W, et al. Outcomes, health-care resources use, and costs of endoscopic removal of metallic airway stents. CHEST.2010;138(2):350-356.

[xxx] Zakaluzny SA, Lane JD, Mair EA. Complications of tracheobronchial airway stents. Otolaryngol Head Neck Surg. 2003 Apr;128(4):478-88.

[xxxi] Goenka MK, Gupta NM, Kochhar R, Rungta U, Vaiphei K, Nagi B, Suri S. Mediastinal fibrosis: an unusual cause of esophageal stricture. J Clin Gastroenterol. 1995 Jun;20(4):331-3.

[xxxii] Zane T. Hammoud, MDa,*, Anthony S. Rose, MDb, Chadi A. Hage, MDb, Kenneth S. Knox, MDb, Karen Rieger, MDc, Kenneth A. Kesler, MD. Surgical Management of Pulmonary and Mediastinal Sequelae of Histoplasmosis: A Challenging Spectrum. Ann Thorac Surg 2009;88:399-403.

[xxxiii] Monroe, Burt L. Jr. and Cronholm, Lois S. Environmental and Health Studies of Kentucky Blackbird Roosts. (1976). Bird Control Seminars Proceedings. Paper 57. http://digitalcommons.unl.edu/icwdmbirdcontrol/57

[xxxiv] Meredith E. Pugh, MD; and James E. Loyd, MD. Fibrosing Mediastinitis: Causes, Diagnosis, and Treatment. PCCSU Article | 01.15.09.

Society of Interventional Radiology. 2012.

National Center for Biotechnology Information, U.S. National Library of Medicine, Bethesda MD.

Society for Vascular Surgery. Chicago, IL http://www.vascularweb.org/vascularhealth/Pages/ct-angiography.aspx. 2012.

David C. Dugdale, III, MD, Professor of Medicine, Division of General Medicine, Department of Medicine, University of Washington School of Medicine; and Stuart I. Henochowicz, MD, FACP, Associate Clinical Professor of Medicine, Division of Allergy, Immunology, and Rheumatology, Georgetown University Medical School. Also reviewed by David Zieve, MD, MHA, Medical Director, A.D.A.M., Inc.

The American Heritage® Medical Dictionary Copyright © 2007, 2004 by Houghton Mifflin Company. Published by Houghton Mifflin Company.

http://picclinenursing.com/about.html

National Center for Biotechnology Information, U.S. National Library of Medicine, Bethesda MD.

ABOUT THE AUTHOR

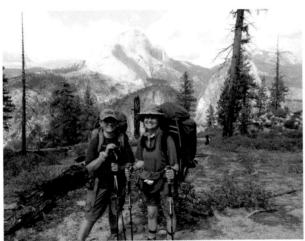

The author (left) and her partner Monica on their quest to conquer Half Dome in Yosemite National Park, CA.

TJ Askren has been a critical care/emergency RN for 27 years. She grew up in the Ohio Valley and was diagnosed with histo-FM in 1999. She is the author of the novel, GROWING WISHBONES, and has published short stories in *Common Lives* and *Frighten the Horses*. She now lives in Ashland, Oregon with her partner and two felines.

www.tjaskren.net

Made in the USA
Middletown, DE
01 March 2023